Activities & Assessment Manual

Third Edition

Jerome E. Kotecki
Ball State University
Muncie, Indiana

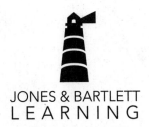

JONES & BARTLETT
LEARNING

World Headquarters
Jones & Bartlett Learning
40 Tall Pine Drive
Sudbury, MA 01776
978-443-5000
info@jblearning.com
www.jblearning.com

Jones & Bartlett Learning Canada
6339 Ormindale Way
Mississauga, Ontario L5V 1J2
Canada

Jones & Bartlett Learning International
Barb House, Barb Mews
London W6 7PA
United Kingdom

Jones & Bartlett Learning books and products are available through most bookstores and online booksellers. To contact Jones & Bartlett Learning directly, call 800-832-0034, fax 978-443-8000, or visit our website, www.jblearning.com.

Substantial discounts on bulk quantities of Jones & Bartlett Learning publications are available to corporations, professional associations, and other qualified organizations. For details and specific discount information, contact the special sales department at Jones & Bartlett Learning via the above contact information or send an email to specialsales@jblearning.com.

The author, editor, and publisher have made every effort to provide accurate information. However, they are not responsible for errors, omissions, or for any outcomes related to the use of the contents of this book and take no responsibility for the use of the products and procedures described. Treatments and side effects described in this book may not be applicable to all people; likewise, some people may require a dose or experience a side effect that is not described herein. Drugs and medical devices are discussed that may have limited availability controlled by the Food and Drug Administration (FDA) for use only in a research study or clinical trial. Research, clinical practice, and government regulations often change the accepted standard in this field. When consideration is being given to use of any drug in the clinical setting, the health care provider or reader is responsible for determining FDA status of the drug, reading the package insert, and reviewing prescribing information for the most up-to-date recommendations on dose, precautions, and contraindications, and determining the appropriate usage for the product. This is especially important in the case of drugs that are new or seldom used.

Production Credits
Publisher, Higher Education: Cathleen Sether
Acquisitions Editor: Shoshanna Goldberg
Senior Associate Editor: Amy L. Bloom
Senior Editorial Assistant: Kyle Hoover
Production Manager: Julie Champagne Bolduc
Production Editor: Jessica Steele Newfell
Associate Marketing Manager: Jody Sullivan
Composition: Glyph International
Cover Design: Kate Ternullo
Cover Images: © Peter Hurley Studio/Chicago
Printing and Binding: Courier Stoughton
Cover Printing: Courier Stoughton

ISBN-13: 978-0-7637-9387-6

6048
Printed in the United States of America
14 13 12 11 10   10 9 8 7 6 5 4 3 2 1

Contents

Preface

This manual provides a practical framework for you to individually apply the concepts outlined in *Physical Activity and Health: An Interactive Approach, Third Edition*. An important step in applying this knowledge is starting with a baseline assessment of your current health status, fitness status, and daily habits. To assist, I have put together more than 70 science-based health and fitness activities and assessments that examine your current status and measure what you are doing now. Completing each activity and assessment will help you identify the aspects of your personal behavior that with modification can improve your overall health.

Your instructor will provide directions indicating which activities and assessments are required assignments and the order and date(s) in which they are due. Each activity and assessment is self-explanatory. I encourage you to complete sections that are not required—now or in the future—on your own to fully recognize your areas of strength and your opportunities for improvement. By identifying areas needing improvement, you will be better able to set personal goals that allow for health enhancement.

To reach your personal goals, it helps to have a map to know where you are heading, the best way to get there, and the ways to travel without getting lost or running into detours. The "Ready, Set, Goals!" activity beginning on page 21 and the Self-Contract activity on page 31 provide such a map. These activities are tailored to the specific stages of readiness to change behavior you read about in Chapter 2. These activities chart a path that puts you in control of your behavior and allow you to decide what to do and how and when to do it.

Finally, I know that completing this manual will provide you with many opportunities for individual reflection as it relates to the management of your health. Self-reflecting on the way you are living will better allow your actions to come naturally into alignment with your sense of what is best for you to create health and happiness.

Name: _____ Course Number: _____

Section: _____ Date: _____

Healthstyle: A Self-Test

Directions: Answer the following questions regarding each dimension of health. Indicate how often you think the statements describe you using the scale below.

1 = Rarely, if ever
2 = Sometimes
3 = Most of the time
4 = Always

Physical Health

1. I accumulate at least 150 minutes (2 hours and 30 minutes) of moderate-intensity aerobic activity or 75 minutes (1 hour and 15 minutes) of vigorous-intensity aerobic activity every week or an equivalent mix of moderate- and vigorous-intensity aerobic activity.   1 2 3 4

2. I include muscle-strengthening activities on 2 or more days a week that work all major muscle groups (legs, hips, back, abdomen, chest, shoulders, and arms).   1 2 3 4

3. I maintain a healthy body weight, which includes evaluating my waist circumference periodically to ensure that fat is not accumulating around my waist.   1 2 3 4

4. I consume a variety of fruits and vegetables each day. In particular, I select from all five vegetable subgroups—dark green, orange, legumes, starchy vegetables, and other vegetables—several times a week.   1 2 3 4

5. I choose my dietary fats wisely by consuming less than 10 percent of my daily calories from saturated fatty acids and less than 300 milligrams per day of cholesterol and keep trans fatty acid consumption below 2 grams daily while eating more monounsaturated and polyunsaturated fats and oils.   1 2 3 4

6. I avoid smoking cigarettes.   1 2 3 4

7. If I choose to drink alcohol, I do so in moderation.   1 2 3 4

8. I have regular check-ups and age-appropriate health screenings completed by health care providers to identify potential health problems early.   1 2 3 4

9. I regularly take steps to avoid injuries (e.g., wearing a safety belt while riding in a car, wearing a helmet while riding a bike).   1 2 3 4

10. I get between 7–9 hours of sleep most nights.   1 2 3 4

1 = Rarely, if ever
2 = Sometimes
3 = Most of the time
4 = Always

Social Health

1. When I meet people, I feel good about the impression I make on them.   1 2 3 4

2. I am open, honest, and get along well with other people.   1 2 3 4

3. I participate in a wide variety of social activities and enjoy being with people who are different from me.   1 2 3 4

4. I try to be a "better person" and work on behaviors that have caused problems in my interactions with others.   1 2 3 4

5. I get along well with the members of my family.   1 2 3 4

6. I am a good listener.   1 2 3 4

7. I am open and accessible to a loving and responsible relationship.   1 2 3 4

8. I have someone I can talk to about my private feelings.   1 2 3 4

9. I consider the feelings of others and do not act in hurtful or selfish ways.   1 2 3 4

10. I consider how what I say might be perceived by others before I speak.   1 2 3 4

Emotional Health

1. I find it easy to laugh about things that happen in my life.   1 2 3 4

2. I avoid using alcohol as a means of helping me forget my problems.   1 2 3 4

3. I can express my feelings without feeling silly.   1 2 3 4

4. When I am angry, I try to let others know in nonconfrontational and and nonhurtful ways.   1 2 3 4

5. I am not a chronic worrier and do not tend to be suspicious of others.   1 2 3 4

6. I recognize when I am stressed and take steps to relax through exercise, quiet time, or other activities.   1 2 3 4

7. I feel good about myself and believe others like me for who I am.   1 2 3 4

8. When I am upset, I talk to others and actively try to work through my problems.   1 2 3 4

9. I am flexible and adapt or adjust to change in a positive way.   1 2 3 4

10. My friends regard me as a stable, emotionally well-adjusted person.   1 2 3 4

Healthstyle: A Self-Test

Environmental Health

1. I am concerned about environmental pollution and actively try to preserve and protect natural resources.   1 2 3 4

2. I report people who intentionally hurt the environment.   1 2 3 4

3. I recycle my garbage.   1 2 3 4

4. I reuse plastic and paper bags and tin foil.   1 2 3 4

5. I vote for pro-environment candidates in elections.   1 2 3 4

6. I write my elected leaders about environmental concerns.   1 2 3 4

7. I consider the amount of packing covering a product when I buy groceries.   1 2 3 4

8. I try to buy products that are recyclable.   1 2 3 4

9. I use both sides of the paper when taking class notes or doing assignments.   1 2 3 4

10. I try not to leave the faucet running too long when I brush my teeth, shave, or bathe.   1 2 3 4

Spiritual Health

1. I believe life is a precious gift that should be nurtured.   1 2 3 4

2. I take time to enjoy nature and the beauty around me.   1 2 3 4

3. I take time alone to think about what's important in life— who I am, what I value, where I fit in, and where I'm going.   1 2 3 4

4. I have faith in a greater power, be it a God-like force, nature, or the connectedness of all living things.   1 2 3 4

5. I engage in acts of caring and good will without expecting something in return.   1 2 3 4

6. I feel sorrow for those who are suffering and try to help them through difficult times.   1 2 3 4

7. I feel confident that I have touched the lives of others in a positive way.   1 2 3 4

8. I work for peace in my interpersonal relationships, in my community, and in the world at large.   1 2 3 4

9. I am content with who I am.   1 2 3 4

10. I go for the gusto and experience life to the fullest.   1 2 3 4

1 = Rarely, if ever
2 = Sometimes
3 = Most of the time
4 = Always

Intellectual Health

1. I think about consequences before I act.   1 2 3 4

2. I learn from my mistakes and try to act differently the next time.   1 2 3 4

3. I follow directions or recommended guidelines and act in ways
likely to keep myself and others safe.   1 2 3 4

4. I consider the alternatives before making decisions.   1 2 3 4

5. I am alert and ready to respond to life's challenges in ways that
reflect thought and sound judgment.   1 2 3 4

6. I do not let my emotions get the better of me when making
decisions.   1 2 3 4

7. I actively learn all I can about products and services before
making decisions.   1 2 3 4

8. I manage my time well rather than let time manage me.   1 2 3 4

9. My friends and family trust my judgment.   1 2 3 4

10. I think about my self-talk (the things I tell myself) and then
examine the evidence to see if my perception and feelings are sound.   1 2 3 4

Occupational Health

1. I am happy with my career choice.   1 2 3 4

2. I look forward to working in my career area.   1 2 3 4

3. The job responsibilities/duties of my career choice are consistent
with my values.   1 2 3 4

4. The payoffs/advantages in my career choice are consistent with
my values.   1 2 3 4

5. I am happy with the balance between my work time and leisure time.   1 2 3 4

6. I am happy with the amount of control I have in my work.   1 2 3 4

7. My work gives me personal satisfaction and stimulation.   1 2 3 4

8. I am happy with the professional/personal growth provided by my job.   1 2 3 4

9. I feel my job allows me to make a difference in the world.   1 2 3 4

10. My job contributes positively to my overall well-being.   1 2 3 4

Healthstyle: A Self-Test

Personal Checklist

Now total your scores in each of the health dimensions and compare them to the ideal scores. Which areas do you need to work on?

	Ideal Score	Your Score
Physical health	40	_____
Social health	40	_____
Emotional health	40	_____
Environmental health	40	_____
Spiritual health	40	_____
Intellectual health	40	_____
Occupational health	40	_____

What Your Scores Mean

Scores of 35–40 points: Excellent. Your answers show that you are aware of the importance of this area to your health. More important, you are putting your knowledge to work for you by practicing good health habits. As long as you continue to do so, this area should not pose a serious health risk. It's likely that you are setting an example for your family and friends to follow. Although you reported a very high score on this part of the assessment, you may want to consider areas where your scores could be improved.

Scores of 30–34 points: Your health practices in this area are good, but there is room for improvement. Look again at the items you answered that scored one or two points. What changes could you make to improve your score? Even a small change in behavior can often help you achieve better health.

Scores of 20–29 points: Your health practices need improvement. Find information on how you could change these behaviors. Perhaps you need help deciding how to make the changes you desire. Assistance is available in this book, from your professor, and from resources on your campus.

Scores of 19 and lower: Your health practices need serious improvement and you may be taking unnecessary risks with your health. Perhaps you are not aware of the risks and what to do about them. In the textbook you will find the information you need to help improve your scores and your health.

Source: Adapted and modified from *Healthstyle: A Self-Test,* by USDHHS Publication Number (PHS) 8150155.

Name: _____ Course Number: _____

Section: _____ Date: _____

Family Health History

Being aware of your family's health history, especially which relatives had or have serious chronic diseases or inherited conditions, can help you and your physician assess your risk of such diseases or conditions. As a result of having this information, you can make choices concerning your lifestyle now that may reduce the likelihood of developing these health problems in the future.

To compile your personal health history and design a health history diagram, start with your own health and that of your brothers and sisters. Then indicate health conditions that affect your mother and father and their brothers and sisters. After completing health information for that generation, collect information about your grandparents' health. You may be aware of some family members' health problems, such as heart disease, obesity, drug addiction, or mental health conditions. In other instances, however, you will need to speak with your relatives to determine whether they have or had diseases or conditions such as prostate or breast cancer, diabetes, hypertension, liver disease, and so on. If you are adopted or cannot find information about individual family members, you may have to leave blanks.

A sample family health history diagram is shown in this assessment. Note that it has spaces for a person to fill in his or her personal health and the health of siblings, parents, aunts, uncles, and grandparents. Of course, your diagram will reflect your family's makeup. After developing your personal health history diagram, answer the following questions.

1. If a particular disease or condition occurs repeatedly in your family, it may be the result of inherited and/or lifestyle factors that are common within your family. Such repeated occurrences may indicate that your risk of the disease or condition is greater than average. Which serious health problems occur more than once in your family health history?

_____

_____

_____

2. Which diseases or conditions in your family history do you think are related to lifestyle practices, such as food choices, lack of regular physical activity, or smoking?

_____

_____

_____

3. Are you aware of actions you can take that may reduce your risk of developing the health problems that often affect or have affected members of your family? If so, list those actions.

_____

_____

_____

4. The course of many diseases and conditions is influenced by lifestyle factors. Your physician can help you determine such factors. Therefore, consider discussing your family health history with your physician. Your physician can also provide advice concerning steps you can take to reduce your risk of developing the health problems that affect or have affected members of your family.

_____

_____

_____

Family Health History Example

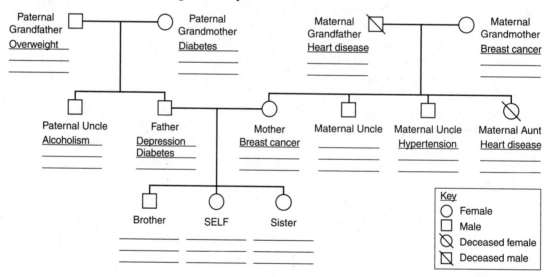

Family Health History

Name: _____ Course Number: _____

Section: _____ Date: _____

Defining Physical Activity and Health

You have had the opportunity to review several definitions regarding physical activity and health. Each person, however, defines physical activity and health according to his or her own values, goals, interests, and other factors that make that person unique. Respond to the following questions based on your personal definition of physical activity and health.

1. What is your personal definition of physical activity?

_____

_____

2. What is your personal definition of health?

_____

_____

3. Are there any similarities in these two definitions?

_____

_____

4. What aspects of your lifestyle reflect your definition of physical activity?

_____

_____

5. What aspects of your lifestyle reflect your definition of health?

_____

_____

6. What aspects of your lifestyle conflict with your definition of physical activity?

_____

_____

7. What aspects of your lifestyle conflict with your definition of health?

_____

_____

8. Describe three actions you plan to take that support your personal definition of physical activity and health.

_____

_____

_____

Source: Adapted from D. A. Birch and M. J. Cleary. (1996). *Managing Your Health: Assessment and Action.* Sudbury, MA: Jones & Bartlett.

Defining Physical Activity and Health

Name: _____ Course Number: _____

Section: _____ Date: _____

Barriers to Being Active Quiz

Directions: Listed below are reasons that people give to describe why they do not get as much physical activity as they think they should. Please read each statement and indicate how likely you are to say each of the following statements:

3 = Very likely
2 = Somewhat likely
1 = Somewhat unlikely
0 = Very unlikely

How Likely Are You to Say . . .

1. My day is so busy now, I just don't think I can make the time to include physical activity in my regular schedule. 3 2 1 0

2. None of my family members or friends like to do anything active, so I don't have a chance to exercise. 3 2 1 0

3. I'm just too tired after work to get any exercise. 3 2 1 0

4. I've been thinking about getting more exercise, but I just can't seem to get started. 3 2 1 0

5. I'm getting older so exercise can be risky. 3 2 1 0

6. I don't get enough exercise because I have never learned the skills for any sport. 3 2 1 0

7. I don't have access to jogging trails, swimming pools, bike paths, etc. 3 2 1 0

8. Physical activity takes too much time away from other commitments—leisure time, work, family, etc. 3 2 1 0

9. I'm embarrassed about how I will look when I exercise with others. 3 2 1 0

10. I don't get enough sleep as it is. I just couldn't get up early or stay up late to get some exercise. 3 2 1 0

11. It's easier for me to find excuses not to exercise than to go out to do something. 3 2 1 0

12. I know of too many people who have hurt themselves by overdoing it with exercise. 3 2 1 0

13. I really can't see learning a new sport at my age.   3 2 1 0

14. It's just too expensive. You have to take a class or join a club or buy the right equipment.   3 2 1 0

15. My free times during the day are too short to include exercise.   3 2 1 0

16. My usual social activities with family or friends do not include physical activity.   3 2 1 0

17. I'm too tired during the week and I need the weekend to catch up on my rest.   3 2 1 0

18. I want to get more exercise, but I just can't seem to make myself stick to anything.   3 2 1 0

19. I'm afraid I might injure myself or have a heart attack.   3 2 1 0

20. I'm not good enough at any physical activity to make it fun.   3 2 1 0

21. If we had exercise facilities and showers at work, then I would be more likely to exercise.   3 2 1 0

Follow these instructions to score yourself:

- Enter the circled number in the spaces provided, putting together the number for statement 1 on line 1, statement 2 on line 2, and so on.

- Add the three scores on each line. Your barriers to physical activity fall into one or more of seven categories: lack of time, social influences, lack of energy, lack of willpower, fear of injury, lack of skill, and lack of resources. A score of 5 or higher in any category shows that this is an important barrier for you to overcome.

_____ + _____ + _____ = _____
 1   8   15   Lack of time

_____ + _____ + _____ = _____
 2   9   16   Social influence

_____ + _____ + _____ = _____
 3   10   17   Lack of energy

_____ + _____ + _____ = _____
 4   11   18   Lack of willpower

_____ + _____ + _____ = _____
 5   12   19   Fear of injury

_____ + _____ + _____ = _____
 6   13   20   Lack of skill

_____ + _____ + _____ = _____
 7   14   21   Lack of resources

Suggestions for Overcoming Physical Activity Barriers

Lack of Time

- Identify available time slots. Monitor your daily activities for one week. Identify at least three 30-minute time slots you could use for physical activity.

- Add physical activity to your daily routine. For example, walk or ride your bike to work or shopping, organize school activities around physical activity, walk the dog, exercise while you watch TV, park farther away from your destination, etc.

- Make time for physical activity. For example, walk, jog, or swim during your lunch hour, or take fitness breaks instead of coffee breaks.

- Select activities requiring minimal time, such as walking, jogging, or stairclimbing.

Social Influence

- Explain your interest in physical activity to friends and family. Ask them to support your efforts.

- Invite friends and family members to exercise with you. Plan social activities involving exercise.

- Develop new friendships with physically active people. Join a group, such as the YMCA or a hiking club.

Lack of Energy

- Schedule physical activity for times in the day or week when you feel energetic.

- Convince yourself that if you give it a chance, physical activity will increase your energy level; then try it.

Lack of Motivation

- Plan ahead. Make physical activity a regular part of your daily or weekly schedule and write it on your calendar.

- Invite a friend to exercise with you on a regular basis and write it on both your calendars.

- Join an exercise group or class.

Fear of Injury

- Learn how to warm up and cool down to prevent injury.

- Learn how to exercise appropriately considering your age, fitness level, skill level, and health status.

- Choose activities involving minimum risk.

Lack of Skill

- Select activities requiring no new skills, such as walking, climbing stairs, or jogging.

- Exercise with friends who are at the same skill level as you are.

- Find a friend who is willing to teach you some new skills.

- Take a class to develop new skills.

Lack of Resources

- Select activities that require minimal facilities or equipment, such as walking, jogging, jumping rope, or calisthenics.

- Identify inexpensive, convenient resources available in your community (community education programs, park and recreation programs, worksite programs, etc.).

Weather Conditions

- Develop a set of regular activities that are always available regardless of weather (indoor cycling, aerobic dance, indoor swimming, calisthenics, stair climbing, rope skipping, mall walking, dancing, gymnasium games, etc.).

- Look on outdoor activities that depend on weather conditions (cross-country skiing, outdoor swimming, outdoor tennis, etc.) as "bonuses"—extra activities possible when weather and circumstances permit.

Travel

- Put a jumprope in your suitcase and jump rope.

- Walk the halls and climb the stairs in hotels.

- Stay in places with swimming pools or exercise facilities.

- Join the YMCA or YWCA (ask about reciprocal membership agreements).

- Visit the local shopping mall and walk for half an hour or more.

- Bring a small tape recorder and your favorite aerobic exercise tape.

Family Obligations

- Trade babysitting time with a friend, neighbor, or family member who also has small children.

- Exercise with the kids—go for a walk together, play tag or other running games, get an aerobic dance or exercise tape for kids (there are several on the market) and exercise together. You can spend time together and still get your exercise.

- Hire a babysitter and look at the cost as a worthwhile investment in your physical and mental health.

- Jump rope, do calisthenics, ride a stationary bicycle, or use other home gym equipment while the kids are busy playing or sleeping.

- Try to exercise when the kids are not around (e.g., during school hours or their nap time).

- Encourage exercise facilities to provide child care services.

Retirement Years

- Look upon your retirement as an opportunity to become more active instead of less. Spend more time gardening, walking the dog, and playing with your grandchildren. Children with short legs and grandparents with slower gaits are often great walking partners.

- Learn a new skill you've always been interested in, such as ballroom dancing, square dancing, or swimming.

- Now that you have the time, make regular physical activity a part of every day. Go for a walk every morning or every evening before dinner. Treat yourself to an exercycle and ride every day while reading a favorite book or magazine.

Source: Content taken from *Promoting Physical Activity: A Guide for Community Action* (USDHHS, 1999).

Chapter 1: Critical Thinking Questions

The Physical Activity and Health Connection

1. Are you feeling lethargic and tired, like Susannah? Could it be because of lack of physical activity? If so, what physical activity are you currently doing? If not, what can you do to increase your physical activity? Develop a list of campus events or organizations that involve physical activity (e.g., hiking club, co-ed intramural volleyball, walking club, kick boxing). Investigate several of them to see which one best fits your needs and schedule. Begin adding this activity into your daily or weekly college routine.

2. Using the seven dimensions of health, identify two behaviors you do that would be an example of enhancing each dimension.

3. The morning newspaper headline is "Scientific studies indicate physical activity is important to health and quality of life." The article mentions studies from the *Prestigious International Health and Medicine Journal.* Later that day, you hear a local radio report suggesting that too much physical activity can lead to an instant heart attack, maybe even death. You are bombarded with health messages daily. What is your major source of health information? Television? If so, which shows in particular? Magazines? School? Friends? How carefully do you analyze health information? Do you believe most of what you read about health, or does it depend on the source?

Critical Thinking Questions

Name: _____ Course Number: _____

Section: _____ Date: _____

Stages of Change: Continuous Measure

Directions

Please use the following exercise recommendations when answering the following questions:

According to the recommendation by the *Physical Activity Guidelines for Americans*, "adults need at least 150 minutes (2 hours and 30 minutes) of moderate-intensity aerobic activity or 75 minutes (1 hour and 15 minutes) of vigorous-intensity aerobic activity every week or an equivalent mix of moderate- and vigorous-intensity **and** muscle-strengthening activities on 2 or more days a week that work all major muscle groups (legs, hips, back abdomen, chest, shoulders, and arms)" (USDHHS, 2008).

Please check off all statements that apply to your lifestyle.

1. As far as I'm concerned, I don't need to exercise regularly. _____

2. I have been exercising regularly for a long time and I plan to continue. _____

3. I don't exercise, and right now I don't care. _____

4. I am finally exercising regularly. _____

5. I have been successful at exercising regularly and I plan to continue. _____

6. I am satisfied with being a sedentary person. _____

7. I have been thinking that I might want to start exercising regularly. _____

8. I have started exercising regularly within the last 6 months. _____

9. I could exercise regularly, but I don't plan to. _____

10. Recently, I have started to exercise regularly. _____

11. I don't have the time or energy to exercise regularly right now. _____

12. I have started to exercise regularly, and I plan to continue. _____

13. I have been thinking about whether I will be able to exercise regularly. _____

14. I have set up a day and a time to start exercising regularly within the next few weeks. _____

Reference: U.S. Department of Health and Human Services. (2008). *Physical Activity Guidelines for Americans.* Online: http://www.health.gov/paguidelines/pdf/paguide.pdf.

15. I have managed to keep exercising regularly through the last 6 months. _____

16. I have been thinking that I may want to begin exercising regularly. _____

17. I have arranged with a friend to start exercising regularly within the next few weeks. _____

18. I have completed 6 months of regular exercise. _____

19. I know that regular exercise is worthwhile, but I don't have time for it in the near future. _____

20. I have been calling friends to find someone to start exercising with in the next few weeks. _____

21. I think regular exercise is good, but I can't figure it into my schedule right now. _____

22. I really think I should work on getting started with a regular exercise program in the next 6 months. _____

23. I am preparing to start a regular exercise group in the next few weeks. _____

24. I am aware of the importance of regular exercise, but I can't do it right now. _____

In the box below, circle the numbers that correspond with the numbers of the statements you checked off. For example, if you checked off statement number 17, find and circle 17 in the box below.

Stages of Change:
Precontemplation (nonbelievers in exercise) items: 1, 3, 6, 9
Precontemplation (believers in exercise) items: 11, 19, 21, 24
Contemplation items: 7, 13, 16, 22
Preparation items: 14, 17, 20, 23
Action items: 4, 8, 10, 12
Maintenance items: 2, 5, 15, 18
Source: Cancer Prevention Research Center (CPRC). *Measures. Exercise: Stages of Change—Continuous Measure.*
Online: http://www.uri.edu/research/cprc/Measures/Exercise01.htm.

- What stage of change has the most numbers circled?

- Do you think this is an accurate measure of where you are in regard to increasing physical activity in your life?

Name: _____   Course Number: _____

Section: _____   Date: _____

Ready, Set, Goals!

This section contains four different goal-setting worksheets. The worksheets are tailored to specific stages of readiness to change behavior. Depending on your stage of readiness, your goals will be different.

Precontemplation or Contemplation

Your goal will be to begin thinking about the healthy lifestyle behavior you selected to work on. You will consider the ways you could benefit from practicing the behavior and think about how you could overcome any obstacles that are blocking you from achieving this goal. This worksheet provides a useful tool for weighing the costs and benefits associated with making a change. It also employs visualization as a technique for thinking about change. You are encouraged to eliminate negative "self-talk" ("I'm always so lazy") and replace it with positive "self-talk" ("I didn't work out last week, but I will today").

Preparation

Your goal will be to commit to the decision you made to change your behavior soon. You will do so by setting small, realistic goals and creating a plan to take action.

You will learn to write SMART goals—that is, goals that are *s*pecific, *m*easurable, *a*chievable, *r*elevant, and *t*rackable. For example, instead of setting a goal to "always eat breakfast," set a more realistic and achievable goal: "I will eat breakfast before Spanish class three mornings this week."

Action

Your goal will be to firmly establish the new behavior as a lifelong habit by anticipating problems and preparing to overcome failures, and by rewarding your successes to stay committed.

Maintenance

Your goal will be to stay focused and renew your commitment to the healthy behavior you selected to work on. You will consider new ways to achieve your goals for long-term health and identify ways to prevent the inevitable slip-ups from becoming full-fledged backslides.

These worksheets are adapted from the "wellStage" brochures developed by Health Enhancement Systems, Inc. (hesonline.com) and are used with permission. These tools are effective in changing not only eating and activity behaviors but also other health behaviors. You are welcome to use these behavior change worksheets in your future area of practice with credit given to the source.

PRECONTEMPLATION OR CONTEMPLATION

Assessment Area: _____

Current Behavior: _____

Target Behavior: _____

Your goal is to begin thinking about this healthy lifestyle behavior. You will consider the ways you could benefit from this behavior and think about how you could overcome any obstacles that are preventing you from practicing this behavior.

Step 1

Imagine that a friend or family member was told by his or her doctor to adopt this behavior. What advantages of this behavior would you highlight to motivate your friend or family member? (List at least three.)

_____

_____

_____

What are some things that might get in the way of this person's efforts to implement the target behavior? (List at least two.) What ideas do you have to help your friend or family member overcome these obstacles?

_____

_____

_____

What suggestions would you make to help this person get started? (What is one small, simple thing he or she could do every day?)

_____

_____

Step 2

Now consider your *own* costs and benefits for adopting this behavior. Fill in the grid on the next page. Which is *greater,* the left side—reasons to change—or the right side—reasons to stay the same?

_____ reasons to change _____ reasons to stay the same

What *one* benefit of the new behavior do you think will motivate you the most?

_____

_____

What *one* "cost" or barrier do you think will present the biggest obstacle for you?

_____

_____

Step 3

Being able to visualize performing the desired behavior is an important step in reshaping your beliefs, attitudes, and behaviors. Visualize yourself practicing the target behavior and all the associated preparation and implementation steps and imagine the subsequent feelings of health and confidence. Write down three distinct visual images of different aspects of practicing this behavior. (Examples include shopping, food preparation, and eating behaviors.) Use positive phrases of self-talk.

_____

_____

_____

Step 4

Start to recognize successes you achieve in practicing this behavior, no matter how small. Look over the records you kept. When were you successful in following the desired behavior even a little? Why do you think you were successful?

_____

_____

_____

Were there certain times of day, or situations, that prevented success? If so, what were they, and how might you prepare for these times so you can be more successful?

_____

_____

_____

Lifestyle Behavior Change: Perceived Costs and Benefits

Perceived Cost of Continuing Current Lifestyle Behavior *Why should I change? How is my current behavior hurting me?*	**Perceived Benefit of Continuing Current Lifestyle Behavior** *What do I give up if I change?*
Perceived Benefit of Adopting New Healthful Lifestyle Behavior *How will this new behavior help me?*	**Perceived Cost of Adopting New Healthful Lifestyle Behavior** *How much will this change "cost" or hurt?*

Step 5

Increasing your knowledge of the advantages of practicing this behavior and the disadvantages of failing to do so can help motivate you for change. What one thing can you learn more about?

_____

_____

Step 6

Other people can help or hinder the behavior change process. Identify at least one person who can support your efforts, and list one or more things he or she can do to provide support.

_____

_____

PREPARATION

Assessment Area: _____

Current Behavior: _____

Target Behavior: _____

Your goal is to commit to the decision you have made to change your behavior _soon_. You will do so by setting small, realistic goals and creating a plan to take action.

Step 1

How do you expect to benefit from adopting this behavior?

_____

_____

Which of these reasons is _most_ important to you, and why?

_____

_____

Step 2

What changes will you need to make to achieve the target behavior? In other words, what will you need to do differently to succeed?

_____

_____

Step 3

Set goals to help you practice the target behavior. **SMART** goals have all of the following characteristics:

S (Specific)	Write down precisely what you want to achieve. Don't be vague.
M (Measurable)	Write down amounts, times, days, and any other measurable factors.
A (Achievable)	Your goal should be realistic—something that challenges you to stretch but is not impossible to achieve. Avoid the words *always* and *never*.
R (Relevant)	Your goal should be important to *you*, rather than simply done as an assignment for class.
T (Trackable)	Recording your progress helps you see what you've achieved and is one of the things that results in long-term success.

Write one or two SMART goals that will help you achieve the target behavior:

1. _____

2. _____

Step 4

Commit to take action. Set a start date. Pick a date at least 5 days before this part is due so that you can try out your goals and record the results of your efforts.

Start date: _____

Tell someone what you plan to do. Being accountable to others motivates you and also offers you the support and encouragement of others.

Who did you tell? _____

Signature: _____

Step 5

Track your progress. For 3 days after your start date, keep track of the results of trying to meet your SMART goal(s) on the following chart:

SMART Goals	Dates	Results

Step 6

Evaluate your progress and continue or modify your plan:

_____

_____

_____

_____

ACTION

Assessment Area: _____

Current Behavior: _____

Target Behavior: _____

Your goal is to firmly establish this behavior as a lifelong habit by anticipating problems and preparing to overcome failures, and by rewarding your successes to stay committed.

Step 1

In what ways have you benefited from adopting this behavior?

_____

_____

What motivates you the most to continue practicing this behavior, and why?

_____

_____

Step 2

What are some of the obstacles that you have encountered that make it difficult to consistently practice this behavior? (Common obstacles include stress, lack of time, travel, and boredom.) List each obstacle you encounter (or anticipate encountering), and identify one or more potential solutions to keep this obstacle from getting in your way of achieving your goal.

Obstacles	Solutions

Step 3

Set goals to help you continue to practice the target behavior. **SMART** goals have all of the following characteristics:

S (Specific)	Write down precisely what you want to achieve. Don't be vague.
M (Measurable)	Write down amounts, times, days, and any other measurable factors.
A (Achievable)	Your goal should be realistic—something that challenges you to stretch but is not impossible to achieve. Avoid the words *always* and *never*.
R (Relevant)	Your goal should be important to *you*, rather than simply done as an assignment for class.
T (Trackable)	Recording your progress helps you see what you've achieved and is one of the things that results in long-term success.

Write one or two SMART goals that will help you consistently achieve the target behavior:

1. _____

2. _____

Step 4

Reward your progress. Permanently changing lifestyle behaviors takes patience and consistent positive reinforcement. List several rewards you could give yourself for meeting your goals:

Select a reward for meeting your goal(s) for 3 days: _____

© 2011 Jones & Bartlett Learning

Step 5

Record your progress toward earning your reward. For 3 days, keep track of the results of trying to meet your SMART goal(s) on the following chart:

SMART Goals	Dates	Results

MAINTENANCE

Assessment Area: _____

Current Behavior: _____

Target Behavior: _____

Your goal is to stay focused and renew your commitment to this behavior. You will consider new ways to achieve your goals for long-term health, and identify ways to prevent the inevitable slip-ups from becoming full-fledged backslides.

Step 1

What benefits of practicing this behavior are most important to you, and why?

_____

_____

Step 2

How easy is this behavior to maintain? Is it truly a habit or do you need to expend some effort to do it?

_____

_____

Sometimes you might get off track briefly (but, hopefully, not permanently) and need to recommit yourself to a particular practice. How frequently do you *not* practice this particular behavior and why?

_____

_____

To prepare for these times, list several situations that might cause you to discontinue this behavior more often than once in a while. For each challenging situation, list one or more ideas to stay, or get back, on track.

Challenges	Solutions

Step 3

Try a new approach to achieving your goal (try a new food, a new recipe, a new activity, a change in routine). List at least two new things you could try:

1. _____

2. _____

Step 4

Record when you tried these new approaches and how it went:

New Approaches	Dates	Results

Step 5

If appropriate, consider writing a more challenging goal to achieve. Write your new goal:

_____

_____

_____

Source: B. Mayfield. (2006). *Personal Nutrition Profile,* 2nd ed. Sudbury, MA: Jones & Bartlett, 109–118.

Ready, Set, Goals!

Name: _____ Course Number: _____

Section: _____ Date: _____

Self-Contract

When you commit in writing what you want to accomplish, you increase the likelihood that you will act accordingly within a certain period of time. Eliciting this type of personal commitment has been shown to be one the most important aspects of health behavior change, especially when you share this self-contract with others close to you.

Start date: _____ Finish date: _____

Goal: _____

Motivation (benefits): _____

Identify your current stage of change: _____

Match your current stage of change and other stages you anticipate
progressing through with the appropriate processes of change:

_____   _____

_____   _____

What specific techniques will you use for each of the processes identified above?	
Processes	Specific Techniques
Stage of change on the finish date:	

Mini goals	Date	Reward
_____	_____	_____
_____	_____	_____
_____	_____	_____

I, _____, agree to work toward a healthier lifestyle and
in doing so shall comply with the terms and dates of this contract.

Signature: _____ Date: _____

Witness: _____ Date: _____

Name: _____   Course Number: _____

Section: _____   Date: _____

Chapter 2: Critical Thinking Questions

Understanding and Enhancing Health Behaviors

1. Often, like Kevin, you might not be ready to make a health behavior change, especially if you think your effort will be greater than the benefit of the behavior. List 10 reasons people begin a physical activity program (benefits) and 10 reasons people do not begin a physical activity program (barriers). Put an *L* next to the benefits that are long term and a *B* next to those that are short term. Turning to the barriers, indicate which you have control over and which you do not. Do the barriers seem to outweigh the benefits? This time focus on short-term benefits and on barriers over which you have control. Does this change the picture?

2. As a friend, housemate, fraternity brother, or sorority sister, what role(s) can you play in supporting someone who is beginning a physical activity program? In analyzing your role, be aware of things you might do that would deter your friend from beginning or maintaining a physical activity program. Avoid those behaviors.

_____

_____

_____

_____

_____

_____

_____

_____

_____

_____

_____

_____

_____

_____

_____

_____

Name: _____ Course Number: _____

Section: _____ Date: _____

PAR-Q and You: A Questionnaire for People Aged 15 to 69

Regular physical activity is fun and healthy, and more people are starting to become more active every day. Being more active is safe for most people. However, some people should check with their doctor before they start becoming much more physically active.

If you are planning to become much more physically active, start by answering the following seven questions.

If you are between the ages of 15 and 69, the PAR-Q will tell you if you should check with your doctor before you start. If you are older than 69 years of age, and you are not used to being very active, check with your doctor. Common sense is your best guide when you answer these questions. Please read the questions carefully and answer each one honestly: Check *yes* or *no*.

Yes   No

____ ____ **1.** Has your doctor ever said that you have a heart condition *and* that you should only do physical activity recommended by a doctor?

____ ____ **2.** Do you feel pain in your chest when you do physical activity?

____ ____ **3.** In the past month, have you had chest pain when you were not doing physical activity?

____ ____ **4.** Do you lose your balance because of dizziness or do you ever lose consciousness?

____ ____ **5.** Do you have a bone or joint problem (e.g., back, knee, hip) that could be made worse by a change in your physical activity?

____ ____ **6.** Is your doctor currently prescribing drugs (e.g., water pills) for your blood pressure or heart condition?

____ ____ **7.** Do you know of *any other reason* why you should not do physical activity?

If You Answered YES to One or More Questions

Talk with your doctor by phone or in person *before* you start becoming much more physically active or *before* you have a fitness appraisal. Tell your doctor about the PAR-Q and which questions you answered YES.

- You may be able to do any activity you want—as long as you start slowly and build up gradually. Or, you may need to restrict your activities to those that are safe for you. Talk with your doctor about the kinds of activities in which you wish to participate and follow the doctor's advice.

- Find out which community programs are safe and helpful for you.

Delay Becoming Much More Active

- If you are not feeling well because of a temporary illness such as a cold or a fever—wait until you feel better; or

- If you are or may be pregnant—talk to your doctor before you start becoming more active.

If You Answered NO to All Questions

If you answered NO honestly to *all* PAR-Q questions, you can be reasonably sure that you can:

- Start becoming much more physically active—begin slowly and build up gradually. This is the safest and easiest way to go.

- Take part in a fitness appraisal—this is an excellent way to determine your basic fitness so that you can plan the best way for you to live actively. It is also highly recommended that you have your blood pressure evaluated. If your reading is over 144/94 mm Hg, talk with your doctor before you start becoming much more physically active.

> **Please Note:** If your health changes so that you then answer YES to any of the preceding questions, tell your fitness or health professional. Ask whether you should change your physical activity plan.

Informed Use of the PAR-Q: The Canadian Society for Exercise Physiology, Health Canada, and their agents assume no liability for persons who undertake physical activity, and, if in doubt after completing this questionnaire, consult your doctor prior to physical activity.

> You are encouraged to copy the PAR-Q, but only if you use the entire form.

Note: If the PAR-Q is being given to a person before he or she participates in a physical activity program or a fitness appraisal, this section may be used for legal or administrative purposes.

I have read, understood, and completed this questionnaire. Any questions I had were answered to my full satisfaction.

Name: _____

Signature: _____ Date: _____

Signature of Parent: _____ Witness: _____
or Guardian (for participants under the age of majority)

Source: Physical Activity Readiness Questionnaire (PAR-Q). © 2002. Reprinted with permission from the Canadian Society for Exercise Physiology. Online: http://www.csep.ca/forms.asp.

Medical History Questionnaire

Directions: This questionnaire is designed to provide your exercise and physical activity professional with information necessary to assist you in the development of a physical activity program. It is not designed as a medical screening device. It is strongly suggested that you check with your physician before making any significant changes in your physical activity status.

Name: _____
       LAST NAME   FIRST NAME   MI

Address: _____

_____

_____

Phone number: _____
           HOME   WORK   EXT

Sex: _____ Date of birth: _____ Height: _____ Weight: _____

Name of physician: _____

Physician's address: _____

_____

Physician's phone number: _____

Person to contact in case of emergency: _____

Contact's address: _____

_____

Contact's phone number: _____

Any medications, foods, or other substances to which you are allergic:

_____

_____

When was the last time you had a physical examination? _____

Please list any chronic or serious illnesses you have as diagnosed by your physician.

_____

_____

_____

_____

Please list any operations you may have had.

_____

_____

_____

Please list any hospitalizations lasting more than 1 day that you may have had (other than normal pregnancies for women).

_____

_____

_____

Please list any prescription medications you are currently taking.

_____

_____

_____

Please list any over-the-counter medications you are currently taking.

_____

_____

_____

Have you experienced any of the following symptoms in the past 12 months?

	Yes	No
Fainting, light-headedness, or blackouts	____	____
Dyspnea or trouble breathing	____	____
Unusual difficulty sleeping	____	____
Blurred vision	____	____
Severe headaches or migraines	____	____
Chronic coughing	____	____
Slurring or loss of speech	____	____
Unusual nervousness or anxiety	____	____
Unusual heartbeats, skipped beats, or palpitations	____	____
Sudden tingling, numbness, or loss of sensation	____	____
Cold feet and hands in warm weather	____	____
Swelling of the feet and/or ankles	____	____
Pains or cramps in the legs	____	____
Pain or discomfort in the chest	____	____
Pressure or heaviness in your chest	____	____

Has a physician ever told you that you have any of the following conditions?

	Yes	No
High blood pressure	____	____
Diabetes	____	____
High cholesterol	____	____
High triglycerides	____	____
Heart attack	____	____
Stroke	____	____
Arteriosclerosis	____	____
Heart murmur	____	____
Angina	____	____
Rheumatic fever	____	____
Aneurysm	____	____
Cancer	____	____
Abnormal ECG	____	____
Emphysema	____	____
Epilepsy	____	____
Arthritis	____	____

Has any member of your immediate family (parents, brothers, sisters, children, grandparents) ever been treated for, or died from, any of the following conditions?

	Yes	No
Diabetes	_____	_____
Heart disease	_____	_____
Stroke	_____	_____
High blood pressure	_____	_____
Do you smoke tobacco products?	_____	_____
If yes, how many per day? _____		

Chapter 3: Critical Thinking Questions

Principles of Physical Fitness Development

1. Explain the differences between health-related fitness and skill-related fitness.

2. There are several scientific fitness principles (overload, progression, specificity, reversibility, recovery, individual differences) that you must adhere to in order to develop an effective physical activity program. Select three different principles and explain them.

3. You can use the FITT formula to help you determine how much exercise is enough for you to build fitness safely and effectively. What does FITT stand for?

_____

_____

_____

_____

_____

_____

_____

_____

_____

_____

_____

_____

_____

_____

_____

_____

_____

_____

Critical Thinking Questions

Name: _____ Course Number: _____

Section: _____ Date: _____

Finding Your Pulse and Target Heart Rate

Finding Your Pulse

Directions: You will need a stopwatch, a digital watch, or a watch with a second hand to take your pulse. Your pulse can be located at several places on your body. The two most common locations are the carotid pulse and the radial pulse.

To Find Your Carotid Pulse

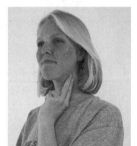

- Turn your head to one side.
- Feel the point at your neck where the large muscle and tendon stick out when your head is turned.
- Slide the fleshy part of your index, middle, and ring fingers along this tendon until you are on a level equal with your Adam's apple.
- Feel for the pulse. Readjust your fingers if necessary. Don't press too hard because this might alter the pulse.
- Count the number of pulses you feel for 60 seconds. This number represents your heart rate in beats per minute. If you are rushed for time, you could count the number of pulses you feel in 15 seconds and multiply this number by 4. Remember, however, that it is more accurate to take a full 60-second count if possible.

To Find Your Radial Pulse

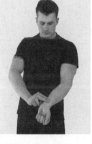

- Hold your forearm out in front of you with your palm facing you.
- Extend your wrist (move the back of your hand toward the back of your forearm).
- At the top portion of your forearm (nearest the thumb) you should see, or at least be able to feel, a tendon just below the wristbone. This is the radial tendon. Your radial pulse can be found just above your radial tendon near the wrist.
- Slide the fleshy part of your index, middle, and ring fingers along this tendon until they are 1 inch from your wrist.
- Feel for the pulse. Readjust your fingers if necessary. Don't press too hard because this might alter the pulse. Count the number of pulses you feel for 60 seconds. This number represents your heart rate in beats per minute.

Finding Your Target Heart Rate

Directions: You can calculate your target heart rate by following these steps. Your target heart rate represents the recommended heart rate zone in which you should attempt to keep your heart rate when training for cardiovascular fitness.

Step 1: $208 - 0.7$ (age) $=$ Estimated maximum heart rate (EMHR)
Step 2: EMHR $-$ Resting heart rate (RHR) $=$ Heart rate reserve (HRR)

_____

_____

Make Sure to Use the Proper Intensity for Your Desired Outcomes

- For those interested in health benefits only, multiply
  HRR $\times$ 40% and HRR $\times$ 55%

  Then add your resting heart rate to these figures to arrive at your target training zone.

  (HRR $\times$ 40%) $+$ RHR $=$ Lower limit of target training zone
  (HRR $\times$ 55%) $+$ RHR $=$ Upper limit of target training zone

- For those interested in optimal health and fitness benefits, multiply
  HRR $\times$ 50% and HRR $\times$ 85%

  Then add your resting heart rate to these figures to arrive at your target training zone.

  (HRR $\times$ 50%) $+$ RHR $=$ Lower limit of target training zone
  (HRR $\times$ 85%) $+$ RHR $=$ Upper limit of target training zone

_____

_____

_____

_____

4.2

Name: _____ Course Number: _____

Section: _____ Date: _____

Calculating Intensity Levels for Cardiorespiratory Endurance Activities

Step 1

Select desired variable to calculate intensity from (this will be determined by what data are available to you).

> *Heart Rate* (go to step 2)
> *Mets* (go to step 15)
> *VO_2 Reserve* (go to step 20)

Heart Rate

Step 2

Select desired intensity level: moderate (proceed to step 3), or vigorous (go to step 9).

Step 3

Use the equation $208 - 0.7$(Age).

___ = ___

Step 4

Subtract your resting heart rate from your answer to step 3.

Step 3 ___ – Resting heart rate ___ = ___

Step 5

Multiply your answer to step 4 by 40 percent.

Step 4 ___ × 0.40 = ___

Step 6

Add your resting heart rate to your answer from step 5. This represents the minimum heart rate you should try to achieve when active.

Resting heart rate ___ + Step 5 ___ = ___

Step 7

Multiply your answer to step 4 by 55 percent.

Step 4 _____ × 0.55 = _____

Step 8

Add your resting heart rate to your answer from step 7. This represents the maximum heart rate you should try to achieve when active.

Resting heart rate _____ + Step 7 _____ = _____

This ends the steps for calculating moderate physical activity intensity from heart rate.

Step 9

Use the equation 208 − 0.7(Age).

Step 10

Subtract your resting heart rate from your answer to step 9.

Step 9 _____ − Resting heart rate _____ = _____

Step 11

Multiply your answer to step 10 by 50%.

Step 10 _____ × 0.50 = _____

Step 12

Add your resting heart rate to your answer from step 11. This represents the minimum heart rate you should try to achieve when active.

Resting heart rate _____ + Step 11 _____ = _____

Step 13

Multiply your answer to step 10 by 85%.

Step 10 _____ × 0.85 = _____

Step 14

Add your resting heart rate to your answer from step 13. This represents the maximum heart rate you should try to achieve when active.

Resting heart rate _____ + Step 13 _____ = _____

This ends the steps for calculating vigorous physical activity intensity from heart rate.

METS

Step 15

Select desired intensity level: moderate (go to step 16), or vigorous (go to step 18).

Step 16

To calculate intensity based on METS, you need to assess your functional aerobic capacity through a graded exercise test.

Step 17

Take 40% and 55% of your maximal MET capacity as determined through a graded exercise test to find the limits for moderate physical activity. For example: if your MET capacity is 10 METS, you should be active at a level of 4 to 5.5 METS.

This ends the steps for calculating moderate physical activity intensity from METS.

Step 18

To calculate intensity based on METS, you need to assess your functional aerobic capacity through a graded exercise test.

Step 19

Take 50% and 85% of your maximal MET capacity as determined through a graded exercise test to find the limits for vigorous physical activity. For example: if your MET capacity is 10 METS, you should be active at a level of 5 to 8.5 METS.

This ends the steps for calculating vigorous physical activity intensity from METS.

VO$_2$ Reserve

Step 20

To calculate moderate intensity based on VO$_2$ reserve, you need to assess your functional aerobic capacity through a graded exercise test. For vigorous intensity calculations, go to step 26.

Step 21

Subtract your resting VO$_2$ (3.5 mL · kg^{-1} · min^{-1}) from your VO$_2$ max score as determined through a graded exercise test to obtain your VO$_2$ reserve.

Step 22

Multiply your VO$_2$ reserve by 40%. For example: if your VO$_2$ reserve is 40 mL · kg^{-1} · min^{-1}, when this figure is multiplied by 40% you get 16 mL · kg^{-1} · min^{-1}.

Step 23

Add your resting VO_2 to your answer from step 22. This represents the minimum VO_2 you should try to achieve when active.

$$3.5 \text{ mL} \cdot \text{kg}^{-1} \cdot \text{min}^{-1} + \text{Step 22} \underline{\hspace{1cm}} = \underline{\hspace{1cm}}$$

Step 24

Multiply your VO_2 reserve by 50%. For example, if your VO_2 reserve is $40 \text{ mL} \cdot \text{kg}^{-1} \cdot \text{min}^{-1}$, when this figure is multiplied by 50% you get $20 \text{ mL} \cdot \text{kg}^{-1} \cdot \text{min}^{-1}$.

Step 25

Add your resting VO_2 to your answer from step 24. This represents the maximum VO_2 you should try to achieve when active.

This ends the steps for calculating moderate physical activity intensity from VO_2 reserve.

Step 26

To calculate vigorous intensity based on VO_2 reserve, you need to assess your functional aerobic capacity through a graded exercise test.

Step 27

Subtract your resting VO_2 ($3.5 \text{ mL} \cdot \text{kg}^{-1} \cdot \text{min}^{-1}$) from your VO_2 max score as determined through a graded exercise test to obtain your VO_2 reserve.

Step 28

Multiply your VO_2 reserve by 50%. For example, if your VO_2 reserve is $40 \text{ mL} \cdot \text{kg}^{-1} \cdot \text{min}^{-1}$, when this figure is multiplied by 50% you get $20 \text{ mL} \cdot \text{kg}^{-1} \cdot \text{min}^{-1}$.

Step 29

Add your resting VO_2 to your answer from step 28. This represents the minimum VO_2 you should try to achieve when active.

$$3.5 \text{ mL} \cdot \text{kg}^{-1} \cdot \text{min}^{-1} + \text{Step 28} \underline{\hspace{1cm}} = \underline{\hspace{1cm}}$$

Step 30

Multiply your VO_2 reserve by 85%. For example, if your VO_2 reserve is $40 \text{ mL} \cdot \text{kg}^{-1} \cdot \text{min}^{-1}$, when this figure is multiplied by 85% you get $34 \text{ ml} \cdot \text{kg}^{-1} \cdot \text{min}^{-1}$.

Step 31

Add your resting VO_2 to your answer from step 29. This represents the maximum VO_2 you should try to achieve when active.

This ends the steps for calculating vigorous physical activity intensity from VO_2 reserve.

Name: _____ Course Number: _____

Section: _____ Date: _____

Rockport Fitness Walking Test™

This activity assesses cardiorespiratory (aerobic) fitness. To perform the test, you need a watch with a second hand to record your time, and you need to wear good walking shoes and loose clothes. You should have your physician's consent before undertaking this exercise test.

Instructions

1. Find a measured track or measure 1 mile using your car's odometer on a level, uninterrupted road.

2. Warm up by walking slowly for 5 minutes.

3. Walk 1 mile as fast as you can, maintaining a steady pace. Note the time that you began walking.

4. When you complete the mile walk, record your time to the nearest second and keep walking at a slower pace. Count your pulse for 15 seconds and multiply by 4, and then record this number. This gives your heart rate per minute after your test walk.

    Heart rate at the end of 1-mile walk: _____ beats per minute

    Time to walk the mile: _____ minutes

5. Remember to stretch once you have cooled down.

6. To find your cardiorespiratory fitness level, refer to the appropriate Rockport Fitness Walking Test™ charts based on your age and sex. These show established fitness norms from the American Heart Association.

    Using your fitness level chart, find your time in minutes and your heart rate per minute. Follow these lines until they meet, and mark this point on your chart. This tells you how fit you are compared to other individuals of your sex and age category.

These charts are based on weights of 170 lb for men and 125 lb for women. If you weigh substantially less, your cardiovascular fitness will be slightly underestimated. Conversely, if you weigh substantially more, your cardiovascular fitness will be slightly overestimated.

How fit you are compared to others of the same age and gender:

Level 5 = high
Level 4 = above average
Level 3 = average
Level 2 = below average
Level 1 = low

Find your fitness level using the Rockport Fitness Walking Test™.

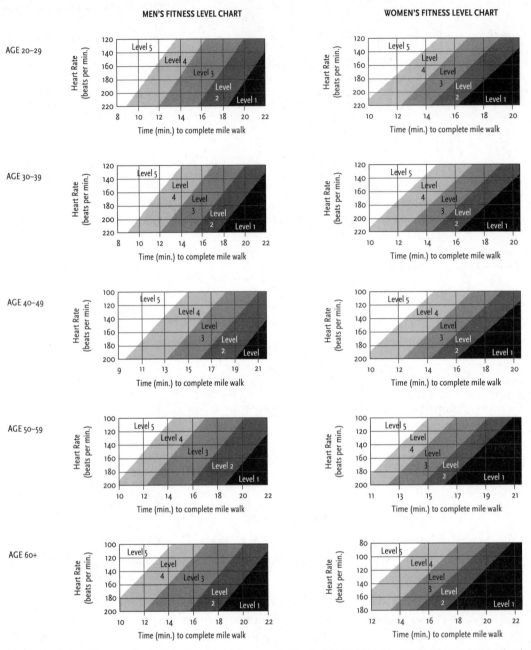

Source: The Rockport Company, Inc., © 1993. *The Rockport Company Walking Test.* The Rockport Company, Inc., Canton, MA. Reprinted with permission of The Rockport Company.

Results and Reflections

Name: _____ Course Number: _____

Section: _____ Date: _____

Chapter 4: Critical Thinking Questions

The Heart of Physical Fitness: Cardiorespiratory Endurance

1. In the vignette, Tammy decided to use the heart rate reserve method to determine her aerobic exercise intensity. What other methods could she have utilized to determine her exercise intensity?

2. Identify four activities in which you are likely to participate that will enhance your cardiorespiratory endurance. Describe how you will incorporate each activity into your daily and weekly routine.

_____

_____

_____

_____

_____

_____

_____

_____

_____

_____

_____

_____

_____

_____

_____

_____

_____

_____

_____

Name: _____ Course Number: _____

Section: _____ Date: _____

Partial Curl-Up Test

Equipment: Mat and Metronome

1. Lie in a supine position with your head resting on a mat, arms straight and parallel to the trunk, palms of the hands in contact with the mat. Have a partner mark a zero line at the tip of your middle finger when in the starting position.

2. Have your partner mark another line 10 cm (4 in.) past the first line in the direction of your feet. Your arms should be fully extended when your fingertips are at the zero mark.

3. Your knees should be bent at a 90-degree angle with your legs hip-width apart. Keep your heels in contact with the mat. Perform the test with your shoes on.

4. Set a metronome to 50 beats per minute.

5. Slowly curl up your upper spine far enough so that the middle finger tips of both hands reach the 10-cm (4-in.) mark. During the curl-up, the palms must remain in contact with the mat. Do not anchor your feet.

6. On the return phase, the shoulder blades and head must contact the mat and the finger tips of both hands should touch the zero mark.

7. Perform the movement in a slow, controlled manner so that the time to perform the lifting and lowering stages of the curl-up is the same at a rate of 25 curl-ups per minute. Breathe normally throughout, exhaling during the upward motion.

8. Perform as many consecutive curl-ups as possible without pausing, to a maximum of 25 in the 1-minute period.

9. Terminate test before 1 minute if you are:

   a. Experiencing undue discomfort.

   b. Unable to maintain the required cadence.

   c. Unable to maintain the proper curl-up technique (e.g., heels come off the floor) over two consecutive repetitions.

10. Record the number of partial curl-ups performed in the 1-minute period.

11. Use the following table to evaluate your score.

Age	Gender	Needs Improvement	Fair	Good	Very Good	Excellent
15–19	Male	≤15	16–20	21–22	23–24	25
	Female	≤11	12–16	17–21	22–24	25
20–29	Male	≤10	11–15	16–20	21–24	25
	Female	≤4	5–13	14–17	18–24	25
30–39	Male	≤10	11–14	15–17	18–24	25
	Female	≤5	6–9	10–18	19–24	25
40–49	Male	≤5	6–12	13–17	18–24	25
	Female	≤3	4–10	11–18	19–24	25
50–59	Male	≤7	8–10	11–16	17–24	25
	Female	≤5	6–9	10–18	19–24	25
60–69	Male	≤5	6–10	11–15	16–24	25
	Female	≤2	3–7	8–16	17–24	25

Source: Canadian Society for Exercise Physiology. (2003). *The Canadian Physical Activity, Fitness & Lifestyle Approach: CSEP-Health & Fitness Program's Health-Related Appraisal & Counseling Strategy,* 3rd ed. Canadian Society for Exercise Physiology. Reprinted with permission.

Name: —————————————————— Course Number: ——————————

Section: —————————————————— Date: ——————————

Push-Up Test for Muscular Endurance

Preparation

- Use a large space on the floor, clear of obstructions.
- Warm-up for 3 to 5 minutes before starting. Give yourself a couple of minutes to recover after warm-up before beginning the test.

Procedure

Men

- Assume the standard position for a push-up, with the body rigid and straight, toes tucked under, and hands about shoulder-width apart and straight under the shoulders.
- Lower the body until the elbows reach 90 degrees. Some prefer to place an object such as a paper cup beneath to touch.
- Return to the starting position with the arms fully extended.
- The most common error is not keeping the back straight and rigid throughout the entire push-up.
- Perform as many push-ups as you can without stopping.
- See the following tables for your fitness level.

Women

Women tend to have less upper body strength and therefore should use the modified push-up position to assess their upper body endurance. The test is performed as follows:

- Directions are the same for women as for men, except that women should perform the test from the bent-knee position. Make sure that your hands are slightly ahead of your shoulders in the up position so that when you are in the down position, your hands are directly under the shoulders.
- Keep the back straight and rigid throughout the entire push-up.
- Perform as many push-ups as you can without stopping.
- See the following tables for your fitness level.

DYNAMIC STRENGTH: 1-Minute Push-Up

	Males Age					
%	**20–29**	**30–39**	**40–49**	**50–59**	**60+**	
99	100	86	64	51	39	
95	62	52	40	39	28	Superior
90	57	46	36	30	26	
85	51	41	34	28	24	
80	47	39	30	25	23	Excellent
75	44	36	29	24	22	
70	41	34	26	21	21	
65	39	31	25	20	20	
60	37	30	24	19	18	Good
55	35	29	22	17	16	
50	33	27	21	15	15	
45	31	25	19	14	12	
40	29	24	18	13	10	Fair
35	27	21	16	11	9	
30	26	20	15	10	8	
25	24	19	13	9.5	7	
20	22	17	11	9	6	Poor
15	19	15	10	7	5	
10	18	13	9	6	4	
5	13	9	5	3	2	Very Poor
n	1045	790	364	172	26	

Total *n* = 2397

These norms are based on worksite wellness program participants.

Source: Reprinted with permission from The Cooper Institute, Dallas, Texas, from *Physical Fitness Assessments and Norms for Adults and Law Enforcement*. Online: http://www.cooperinstitute.org.

DYNAMIC STRENGTH: 1-Minute Full-Body Push-Up*

%	20–29	30–39	40–49	
	Females **Age**			
%	**20–29**	**30–39**	**40–49**	
99	53.0	48.0	23.0	
95	42.0	39.5	20.0	Superior
90	37.0	33.0	18.0	
85	33.0	26.0	17.0	
80	28.0	23.0	15.0	Excellent
75	27.0	19.0	15.0	
70	24.0	18.0	14.0	
65	23.0	16.0	13.0	
60	21.0	15.0	13.0	Good
55	19.0	14.0	11.0	
50	18.0	14.0	11.0	
45	17.0	13.0	10.0	
40	15.0	11.0	9.0	Fair
35	14.0	10.0	8.0	
30	13.0	9.0	7.0	
25	11.0	9.0	7.0	
20	10.0	8.0	6.0	Poor
15	9.0	6.5	5.0	
10	8.0	6.0	4.0	
5	6.0	4.0	1.0	
1	3.0	1.0	0.0	Very Poor

* Full-body push-ups are generally used by law enforcement and public safety organizations.

These norms are based on >1000 female U.S. Army soldiers who were tested in the 1990s by the U.S. Army.

Source: Reprinted with permission from The Cooper Institute, Dallas, Texas, from *Physical Fitness Assessments and Norms for Adults and Law Enforcement*. Online: http://www.cooperinstitute.org.

Name: _____ Course Number: _____

Section: _____ Date: _____

Resistance Training Log

Track and record your muscular strength and endurance progress.

Activity 1: Tracking Your Muscular Endurance

The following charts will help you to track your muscular endurance on different dates. Try to measure yourself at the same time and under the same conditions. These records can provide information as you pursue a physical activity program. Perform the activities in Assessments 5.1 and 5.2 to obtain values and classifications. Record your values below.

Test 1 Date: _____

Assessment technique	Value	Classification
Partial curl-up test		
Push-up test		
Other:		

Test 2 Date: _____

Assessment technique	Value	Classification
Partial curl-up test		
Push-up test		
Other:		

Test 3 Date: _____

Assessment technique	Value	Classification
Partial curl-up test		
Push-up test		
Other:		

Test 4 Date: _____

Assessment technique	Value	Classification
Partial curl-up test		
Push-up test		
Other:		

Activity 2: Resistance Training

Sample of Resistance Exercises

Muscle Group	Training with Weights (free weights or resistance machines)	Without Weights
Chest	Bench press	Push-ups; modified push-ups
Shoulder	Shoulder press	Pull-ups, chin-ups, modified dips
Arm (bicep)	Bicep curl	Arm curl, chin-ups
Arm (tricep)	Tricep curl	Pull-ups, modified dips
Hip/leg	Lunges	Lunges
Leg (thigh)	Half squat	
Leg (calf)	Heel raise	Heel raise

Monitor your workouts by recording the number of sets, repetitions, and the amount of weight.

Muscle group exercises	Date: set × rep / wt	Date: set × rep / wt	Date: set × rep / wt	Date: set × rep / wt	Date: set × rep / wt
	× /	× /	× /	× /	× /
	× /	× /	× /	× /	× /
	× /	× /	× /	× /	× /
	× /	× /	× /	× /	× /
	× /	× /	× /	× /	× /
	× /	× /	× /	× /	× /
	× /	× /	× /	× /	× /
	× /	× /	× /	× /	× /
	× /	× /	× /	× /	× /
	× /	× /	× /	× /	× /

Chapter 5: Critical Thinking Questions

The Power of Resistance Training: Strengthening Your Health

1. List five ways resistance training improves your health.

2. Explain the sliding filament theory of muscle contraction.

3. Explain two differences between slow-twitch and fast-twitch muscle fibers.

4. Explain the differences between static and dynamic resistance-type exercises.

5. Explain the FITT principle as it applies to a resistance training program.

_____

_____

_____

_____

_____

_____

_____

_____

_____

_____

_____

_____

_____

_____

_____

_____

_____

_____

_____

_____

_____

6.1

Name: _____ Course Number: _____

Section: _____ Date: _____

Sit-and-Reach Test

Precautions

1. Warm up.

2. Stop the test if pain occurs.

3. Do not be competitive. Do not perform fast, jerky movements.

4. If any of the following apply, seek medical advice before performing tests:

    a. You are presently suffering from acute back pain.

    b. You are currently receiving treatment for back pain.

    c. You have ever had a surgical operation on your back.

    d. A health care professional told you to never exercise your back.

Procedure

Step 1

Sit on the floor with your legs straight, knees together, and toes pointing upward toward the ceiling.

Step 2

Place one hand over the other. The tips of your two middle fingers should be on top of each other.

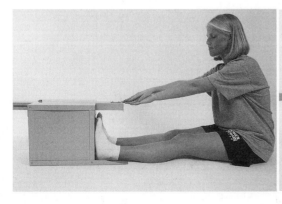 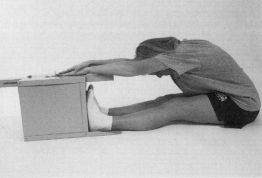

Step 3

Slowly stretch forward without bouncing or jerking. Stop when tightness or discomfort occurs in the back or legs.

Step 4

Repeat this test two more times and record scores.

First attempt   —————— points

Second attempt   —————— points

Third attempt   —————— points

How to score (average of 3 attempts):

Reached well past toes	1 point; excellent
Reached just to toes	2 points; good
Up to 4 inches from toes	3 points; fair
More than 4 inches from toes	4 points; poor

Source: David Imrie. (1988). *Back Power.* Toronto, Canada: Stoddart, 83.

Total points = —————— divided by 3 = —————— points, which is rated as ——————.

Sit-and-Reach Test

Name: _____ Course Number: _____

Section: _____ Date: _____

Stretching Log

Track and record your flexibility and stretching exercises.

Activity 1: Tracking Your Flexibility

Procedure

The following charts will help you to track your flexibility assessment values and the types of stretching exercises you perform each week. The most commonly employed flexibility assessment is the sit-and-reach test you completed in Activity 6.1. Record your scores below. Other joint-specific flexibility assessments are listed to allow you to record your scores.

Test 1 Date: _____

Assessment technique	Value	Classification
Sit-and-reach		
Shoulder		
Thigh		
Calf		
Hamstring		
Groin		
Hip flexors		

Test 2 Date: _____

Assessment technique	Value	Classification
Sit-and-reach		
Shoulder		
Thigh		
Calf		
Hamstring		
Groin		
Hip flexors		

Test 3 Date: _____

Assessment technique	Value	Classification
Sit-and-reach		
Shoulder		
Thigh		
Calf		
Hamstring		
Groin		
Hip flexors		

Test 4 Date: _____

Assessment technique	Value	Classification
Sit-and-reach		
Shoulder		
Thigh		
Calf		
Hamstring		
Groin		
Hip flexors		

Test 5 Date: _____

Assessment technique	Value	Classification
Sit-and-reach		
Shoulder		
Thigh		
Calf		
Hamstring		
Groin		
Hip flexors		

Test 6 Date: _____

Assessment technique	Value	Classification
Sit-and-reach		
Shoulder		
Thigh		
Calf		
Hamstring		
Groin		
Hip flexors		

Stretching Log

Step 1: Select stretching exercises and write them in the left column.

Step 2: Circle the days of each week you stretched.

Exercise	Week of	Week of	Week of
	S M T W Th F Sa	S M T W Th F Sa	S M T W Th F Sa
	S M T W Th F Sa	S M T W Th F Sa	S M T W Th F Sa
	S M T W Th F Sa	S M T W Th F Sa	S M T W Th F Sa
	S M T W Th F Sa	S M T W Th F Sa	S M T W Th F Sa
	S M T W Th F Sa	S M T W Th F Sa	S M T W Th F Sa
	S M T W Th F Sa	S M T W Th F Sa	S M T W Th F Sa
	S M T W Th F Sa	S M T W Th F Sa	S M T W Th F Sa
	S M T W Th F Sa	S M T W Th F Sa	S M T W Th F Sa
	S M T W Th F Sa	S M T W Th F Sa	S M T W Th F Sa
	S M T W Th F Sa	S M T W Th F Sa	S M T W Th F Sa
	S M T W Th F Sa	S M T W Th F Sa	S M T W Th F Sa
	S M T W Th F Sa	S M T W Th F Sa	S M T W Th F Sa

Exercise	Week of	Week of	Week of
	S M T W Th F Sa	S M T W Th F Sa	S M T W Th F Sa
	S M T W Th F Sa	S M T W Th F Sa	S M T W Th F Sa
	S M T W Th F Sa	S M T W Th F Sa	S M T W Th F Sa
	S M T W Th F Sa	S M T W Th F Sa	S M T W Th F Sa
	S M T W Th F Sa	S M T W Th F Sa	S M T W Th F Sa
	S M T W Th F Sa	S M T W Th F Sa	S M T W Th F Sa
	S M T W Th F Sa	S M T W Th F Sa	S M T W Th F Sa
	S M T W Th F Sa	S M T W Th F Sa	S M T W Th F Sa
	S M T W Th F Sa	S M T W Th F Sa	S M T W Th F Sa
	S M T W Th F Sa	S M T W Th F Sa	S M T W Th F Sa
	S M T W Th F Sa	S M T W Th F Sa	S M T W Th F Sa
	S M T W Th F Sa	S M T W Th F Sa	S M T W Th F Sa

Exercise	Week of	Week of	Week of
	S M T W Th F Sa	S M T W Th F Sa	S M T W Th F Sa
	S M T W Th F Sa	S M T W Th F Sa	S M T W Th F Sa
	S M T W Th F Sa	S M T W Th F Sa	S M T W Th F Sa
	S M T W Th F Sa	S M T W Th F Sa	S M T W Th F Sa
	S M T W Th F Sa	S M T W Th F Sa	S M T W Th F Sa
	S M T W Th F Sa	S M T W Th F Sa	S M T W Th F Sa
	S M T W Th F Sa	S M T W Th F Sa	S M T W Th F Sa
	S M T W Th F Sa	S M T W Th F Sa	S M T W Th F Sa
	S M T W Th F Sa	S M T W Th F Sa	S M T W Th F Sa
	S M T W Th F Sa	S M T W Th F Sa	S M T W Th F Sa
	S M T W Th F Sa	S M T W Th F Sa	S M T W Th F Sa
	S M T W Th F Sa	S M T W Th F Sa	S M T W Th F Sa

Exercise	Week of	Week of	Week of
	S M T W Th F Sa	S M T W Th F Sa	S M T W Th F Sa
	S M T W Th F Sa	S M T W Th F Sa	S M T W Th F Sa
	S M T W Th F Sa	S M T W Th F Sa	S M T W Th F Sa
	S M T W Th F Sa	S M T W Th F Sa	S M T W Th F Sa
	S M T W Th F Sa	S M T W Th F Sa	S M T W Th F Sa
	S M T W Th F Sa	S M T W Th F Sa	S M T W Th F Sa
	S M T W Th F Sa	S M T W Th F Sa	S M T W Th F Sa
	S M T W Th F Sa	S M T W Th F Sa	S M T W Th F Sa
	S M T W Th F Sa	S M T W Th F Sa	S M T W Th F Sa
	S M T W Th F Sa	S M T W Th F Sa	S M T W Th F Sa
	S M T W Th F Sa	S M T W Th F Sa	S M T W Th F Sa
	S M T W Th F Sa	S M T W Th F Sa	S M T W Th F Sa

Exercise	Week of	Week of	Week of
	S M T W Th F Sa	S M T W Th F Sa	S M T W Th F Sa
	S M T W Th F Sa	S M T W Th F Sa	S M T W Th F Sa
	S M T W Th F Sa	S M T W Th F Sa	S M T W Th F Sa
	S M T W Th F Sa	S M T W Th F Sa	S M T W Th F Sa
	S M T W Th F Sa	S M T W Th F Sa	S M T W Th F Sa
	S M T W Th F Sa	S M T W Th F Sa	S M T W Th F Sa
	S M T W Th F Sa	S M T W Th F Sa	S M T W Th F Sa
	S M T W Th F Sa	S M T W Th F Sa	S M T W Th F Sa
	S M T W Th F Sa	S M T W Th F Sa	S M T W Th F Sa
	S M T W Th F Sa	S M T W Th F Sa	S M T W Th F Sa
	S M T W Th F Sa	S M T W Th F Sa	S M T W Th F Sa
	S M T W Th F Sa	S M T W Th F Sa	S M T W Th F Sa

Chapter 6: Critical Thinking Questions

Focus on Flexibility: Stretching for Better Health

1. The health benefits of being flexible—the ability to move a joint through its complete range of motion—are many. List three health benefits and how each could enhance your quality of life.

2. Based on your current flexibility program and time commitments, identify three different types of stretching exercises and briefly explain which type you would prefer and why.

3. Many factors influence the amount of flexibility you have at a joint. List two factors over which you have control and whether or not you have taken action on these factors.

_____

_____

_____

_____

_____

_____

_____

_____

_____

_____

_____

_____

_____

_____

_____

_____

_____

Name: _____ Course Number: _____

Section: _____ Date: _____

Part A: Diet and Activity Records

Worksheets are provided in Appendix A of this manual to record your dietary intake and your activities. Select a combination of weekdays and weekend days according to your instructor's directions. Use a new record for each day. The worksheets have been labeled accordingly. Be sure to fill in your name and the date and indicate whether it was a weekday or weekend day at the top of each record. The idea is to get a representative record of intake and expenditure on both typical "workdays" and typical "leisure days." Each day, fill in *both* a diet record and an activity record. This step is important for comparing energy intake and expenditure.

It is essential for you to be complete, accurate, and honest in your record keeping. If the information you record is fictional or inaccurate, you will not learn anything personally valuable from your analysis and the hours you spend on this effort will be a waste of time. You do not get a better grade for "healthier" habits, so don't fake the information to "look better." Take the records with you and log information continuously throughout the day rather than waiting until the end of the day and relying on your memory. Keep track of *everything* you consume and *everything* you do, accurately listing the amounts and times. Using a pencil will allow you to correct mistakes, but be sure it writes dark enough to be readable and photocopy well.

Directions for Completing the Diet Records

The diet record is quite detailed, but the information will prove very useful when you analyze your eating behaviors, and much of the information is recorded only once for each eating event. Each time an eating event occurs, whether it is a meal, a snack, or the consumption of a beverage, record the following information as indicated on the sample diet record:

- What time of day it was, including whether it was a.m. or p.m.

- Whether the event was a meal (M), a snack (S), or a beverage (B).

- How hungry or thirsty you were (record in the column labeled "H"); see the rating scale at the bottom of the worksheet.

- Where you were, such as a cafeteria, restaurant, kitchen table, bedroom, or car (record in the column labeled "Location," and be as specific as you can).

- Whether you were doing any activity while eating (such as driving, watching TV, studying, or talking on the phone).

- If others were present, who (roommates, spouse, friends, and so on), or else write "alone."

- How much time was spent eating/drinking (record in minutes)?

All of this information need be recorded only once for each eating event.

Recording Your Food and Beverage Intake

- In the column labeled "Foods Eaten," record each food and beverage you consumed on a separate line.

- Measure and record the amounts *eaten* using standard units of measurement (e.g., cups, teaspoons, tablespoons, ounces, size of food). The amount you record is the amount you *ate*, not necessarily the amount you were served. *Accurate measurement is critical for your assessment to be valid.*

- Be specific about brand names, types or varieties of food, and preparation (e.g., *Pepperidge Farm whole wheat* bread, *cheddar* cheese, 1% milk, *Del Monte canned* pineapple *in heavy syrup*).

- Don't forget to list extras such as condiments, dressings, gravies, and sauces.

- Record all beverages consumed, including water.

- Record any dietary supplements taken. (You will *not* enter this information into your computer analysis, but will analyze it separately.)

For combination foods, list the components on separate lines.

For example, instead of "1 turkey sub," write 12-inch wheat sub bun, 6 1-ounce slices turkey, 3 leaves lettuce, 3 slices tomato, 2 tablespoons mayonnaise.

Picturing Portions

A *portion* is the amount of food you actually eat. It may be more or less than the standard *serving*, which is the amount listed on food labels and the reference amount listed in food composition tables. As much as possible, measure your food when you keep your diet records. When that is not possible, you can compare the size or amount to common objects:

A *medium* potato is the size of a computer mouse.

A *medium-size* fruit or vegetable is the size of your clenched fist or a tennis ball.

One-half cup of rice, pasta, cereal, or chopped vegetables or fruit is a rounded handful.

One-fourth cup of dried fruit or raisins is the size of a golf ball.

An *average* bagel is the size of a hockey puck.

A pancake or a slice of bread is the size of a compact disk (CD).

A *cup* of fruit is the size of a baseball.

A *cup* of lettuce is four leaves.

Three ounces of cooked meat or poultry is the size of a cassette tape or a deck of cards.

Three ounces of grilled fish is the size of your checkbook.

One ounce of cheese is the size of four dice or two dominoes.

One teaspoon of butter or margarine is the size of a postage stamp.

One tablespoon of salad dressing is the size of a thumb tip.

Two tablespoons of peanut butter is the size of a Ping-Pong ball.

One cup of cooked dry beans is the size of a tennis ball.

One ounce of nuts or small candies is one small handful.

One ounce of chips or pretzels is a large handful.

Recording Measures of Motivators to Eat, Eating More/Less Than Served, and Termination of Eating

- In the column labeled "Reason for Choice," describe *why* you chose each food. Some possible reasons are listed at the bottom of the worksheet, but many others exist.

- Indicate in the column labeled "Helpings" whether you ate less than (−), equal to (0), or more than (+) your *original* helping of that food/beverage.

> The amount of food recorded in the "Food Eaten" column should be the amount eaten, not the amount served. For example, if you measured out one cup, but ate only three-fourths of a cup, list 3/4 cup in the "Food Eaten" column and designate that less was eaten than was served by putting a minus sign (−) in the "Helpings" column.

- The final column, labeled "S," need be filled in only once at the end of each eating event. Indicate your degree of satiation (fullness) using the rating scale provided at the bottom of the worksheet.

Directions for Completing the Activity Records

Record your activities on the same days you keep your diet records. Worksheets are labeled day 1, day 2, day 3, and so on, for this purpose. Be sure to record your name and the date, and indicate whether it was a weekday or weekend day at the top of each worksheet.

- Begin each day with 12 a.m. (midnight) and end with the following midnight.

- Every time you change from one activity to another, record the time you ended the previous activity and started the new one, and describe the type of activity.

- Break down your activity record so that each line is consecutive to cover the 1440 minutes in 24 hours.

- Each time your activity changes, make a new entry.

- Periodically throughout the day, or at the end of the day, fill in the duration and the level of activity columns.

- Record duration in minutes. For example, if you slept from midnight to 7:15 a.m., record 435 minutes.

- At the end of 24 hours, the total time you have recorded must equal 1440 minutes.

You can use the following table to determine your "level of activity." Similar activities have very similar energy expenditures, so they can be grouped together on your activity record if they occurred in the same time period (e.g., reading and typing as part of "studying").

Although activities such as playing computer games or watching television use the same amount of energy as studying, list these activities separately on your activity record so that you have an accurate reflection of how you spend your time. In other words, if you are watching TV and studying at the same time, determine how much time you are doing each activity and record them accordingly. If in your assessment you determine that you are more sedentary than your energy intake allows for, it would be better to cut back on time spent watching TV or playing computer games than on time spent studying.

Basal Metabolism   The energy cost of staying alive (e.g., sleeping, lying motionless).

Sedentary   (0.01 kcal/min/kg) Sitting with little or no body movements (e.g., reading, writing, eating, watching television, driving, sewing).

Light   (0.02 kcal/min/kg) Sitting or standing with some movement of arms and other parts of the body (e.g., preparing food, dishwashing, walking at 2 mi/h, bathing).

Moderate   (0.03 kcal/min/kg) Sitting with vigorous arm movements, or standing with considerable movement (e.g., making beds, mopping, walking at 4 mi/h, warm-up and cooldown exercises, bowling, golfing).

Vigorous   (0.06 kcal/min/kg) Moving body rapidly (e.g., tennis, jogging, weight-lifting, team sports—basketball, baseball, football—but only while playing).

Strenuous   (0.10 kcal/min/kg) Moving body at maximum or near maximum capacity (e.g., swimming laps, running, rope jumping). This level is aerobic activity. Do not include warm-up and cooldown periods.

Examples of diet and activity records are provided on the following pages.

Diet Record Day 1

Name: _____ *Sample* Date: _____ ☐ Weekday
☐ Weekend Day

Eating Behavior Diary

Time of Day	M, S, or B[1]	H[2] (0–3)	Location	Activity While Eating	Others Present	Time Spent Eating	Food Eaten and Quantity (describe preparation, variety, etc., as needed)	Reason for Choice[3]	Helpings (0,–,+)[4]	S[5] (0–3)
7:45 a.m.	M	2	Dining hall	Visiting	Friends	15 min	6 ounces orange juice	Health	0	2
							1 cup Cheerios	Health, habit	–	
							3/4 cup 2% milk	Health, habit	–	
							1/2 toasted bagel	Taste	0	
							1 Tbsp cream cheese	Taste	0	
9:30 a.m.	B	1	Union	Studying	Alone	30	16-ounce Coke	Caffeine	0	2
11:35 a.m.	M	2	McDonald's	Reading paper	Alone	20	Quarter Pounder with cheese	Taste	–	3
							Large French fry	Comfort	0	
							Large Coke	Caffeine	–	
4:15 p.m.	B	2	Swimming pool	Changing clothes	Alone	10	1/2 of 16-ounce water bottle	Thirsty	0	1
5:00 p.m.	B	2	Swimming pool	Changing clothes	Alone	10	1/2 of 16-ounce water bottle	Thirsty	0	1
5:50 p.m.	M	2	Dining hall	Visiting	Friends	30	12 ounces 2% milk	Health, habit	0	2
							12 ounces water	Health	0	
							1 cup tossed salad	Health	0	
							1 ounce grated cheese	Taste, health	0	
							2 Tbsp ranch dressing	Taste	0	

[1] Indicate whether the eating/drinking event was a meal, a snack, or a beverage.

[2] Degree of hunger: 0 = not at all hungry; 1 = slightly hungry; 2 = moderately hungry; 3 = very hungry. If only a beverage was consumed, apply the scale to the degree of thirst.

[3] Reason for food choice: Examples include taste, habit, convenience, health, weight control, hunger, thirst, stress, comfort, offered to me, and so on.

[4] Helpings: 0 = ate all that you were first served but not more; – = ate less than what you were served; + = ate more than you were originally served.

[5] Degree of satiation: 0 = not at all satisfied; 1 = still a little hungry; 2 = satisfied and comfortable; 3 = very full.

Eating Behavior Diary

Time of Day	M, S, or B[1]	H[2] (0–3)	Location	Activity While Eating	Others Present	Time Spent Eating	Food Eaten and Quantity (describe preparation, variety, etc., as needed)	Reason for Choice[3]	Helpings (0,–,+)[4]	S[5] (0–3)
							3" × 3" square of lasagna:	Taste, health	0	
							1.5 ounces lasagna noodles, cooked			
							1 ounce cooked ground beef			
							1.5 ounces cottage cheese			
							4 ounces pasta sauce			
							1 ounce grated mozzarella cheese			
							2 slices garlic bread	Taste, habit	+	
							1 cup soft-serve ice cream	Taste	+	
10 p.m.	S	1	Dorm room	Studying	Alone	5 min	Snickers bar	Taste, habit	0	2
							16-ounce bottle fruit punch	Taste	0	

[1] Indicate whether the eating/drinking event was a meal, a snack, or a beverage.

[2] Degree of hunger: 0 = not at all hungry; 1 = slightly hungry; 2 = moderately hungry; 3 = very hungry. If only a beverage was consumed, apply the scale to the degree of thirst.

[3] Reason for food choice: Examples include taste, habit, convenience, health, weight control, hunger, thirst, stress, comfort, offered to me, and so on.

[4] Helpings: 0 = ate all that you were first served but not more; – = ate less than what you were served; + = ate more than you were originally served.

Activity Record Day 1

Name: _____*Sample*_____ Date: _____

☐ Weekday
☐ Weekend Day

Activity Record

Time of Day	Duration (Minutes)	Description of Activity	Level of Activity
12 – 7:15 a.m.	435	sleeping	basal
7:15 – 7:30	15	showering	light
7:30 – 7:40	10	dressing	light
7:40 – 7:45	5	walking	light
7:45 – 8:00	15	eating breakfast	sedentary
8:00 – 8:15	15	getting ready for class	light
8:15 – 8:30	15	walking to class	moderate
8:30 – 9:20	50	sitting in class	sedentary
9:20 – 9:30	10	walking to Union	moderate
9:30 – 10:20	50	sitting, reading	sedentary
10:20 – 10:30	10	walking to class	moderate
10:30 – 11:20	50	sitting in class	sedentary
11:20 – 11:35	15	walking to McDonald's	moderate
11:35 – 11:55	20	eating lunch	sedentary
11:55 – 12:00	5	walking to store	moderate
12:00 – 12:20	20	shopping for supplies	light
12:20 – 12:30	10	walking to library	moderate
12:30 – 2:20	110	studying	sedentary
2:20 – 2:30	10	walking to class	moderate
2:30 – 3:20	50	sitting in class	sedentary
3:20 – 3:35	15	walking to dorm	moderate
3:35 – 4:00	25	reading mail	sedentary
4:00 – 4:05	5	getting ready to swim	light
4:05 – 4:15	10	walking to swimming pool	moderate
4:15 – 4:25	10	change clothes, shower	light
4:25 – 4:30	5	warm-up swim	moderate
4:30 – 4:50	20	swim laps	strenuous
4:50 – 4:55	5	cooldown swim	moderate

Activity Record

Time of Day	Duration (Minutes)	Description of Activity	Level of Activity
4:55 – 5:15	20	shower and dress	light
5:15 – 5:25	10	walking to dorm	moderate
5:25 – 5:45	20	stand and talk to friends	light
5:45 – 5:50	5	walk to cafeteria	moderate
5:50 – 6:20	30	eat supper	sedentary
6:20 – 7:00	40	read e-mail, surf Internet	sedentary
7:00 – 7:45	45	watch television	sedentary
7:45 – 8:00	15	walk to study session	moderate
8:00 – 9:00	60	attend study session	sedentary
9:00 – 9:15	15	walk to dorm	moderate
9:15 – 11:00	105	studying	sedentary
11:00 – 11:15	15	getting ready for bed	light
11:15 – 12:00	45	sleeping	basal

Total Duration: 1440   (must equal 1440 minutes for the entire 24-hour period)

Name: _____ Course Number: _____

Section: _____ Date: _____

Part B: Diet and Activity Analysis Program Reports

You can use a diet and exercise analysis software program to help you analyze your diet and activity habits, or you can analyze them manually. Follow the directions in the instruction booklet that came with your software program.

As soon as you have completed your diet and activity records, enter your data into the software program. Be careful to enter the data for each day according to the program directions so that your food intake and energy expenditure information will be matched day for day. Print reports that give you information about each day as well as reports that average your intake and expenditure over all the days you kept records. Check your work carefully to be sure that the correct amounts and types of foods and the correct times and types of activities are entered.

Print reports for each day that provide the following information:

- Nutrient intake totals for the day, including total calories, water, protein, carbohydrates, fats, cholesterol, fiber, alcohol, caffeine, vitamins, and minerals. (In the manual, this report will be called "Daily Nutrient Intake.")

  Name of this report in my software program: _____

- The percentage of calories from protein, carbohydrate, and fat; the percentage of fat from various types of fat; and a comparison of the intake for each nutrient to the Dietary Reference Intakes (DRIs). (These data may be included in the same report as the information listed above. In the manual, this report will be called "Daily Nutrient Percent.")

  Name of this report in my software program: _____

- If available, the nutrient breakdown for all foods included in the dietary analysis so that you can identify which foods provide particular nutrients in your diet. (In the manual, this spreadsheet will be called "Nutrient Composition of Foods.")

  Name of this report in my software program: _____

- Energy expenditure information for the activities you performed each day. (In the manual, this report will be called "Daily Energy Expenditure.")

  Name of this report in my software program: _____

Print the following reports as an average of *all* days:

- A report that provides your average nutrient totals for all days, including total calories, water, protein, carbohydrates, fats, cholesterol, fiber, alcohol, caffeine, vitamins, and minerals. (In the manual, this report will be called "Average Nutrient Intake.")

  Name of this report in my software program: _____

- A report that provides your average percentage of calories from protein, carbohydrate, and fat; the percentage of fat from various types of fat; and a comparison of intake for each nutrient to the Dietary Reference Intakes. (These data may be included in the same report as the information listed above. In the manual, this report will be called "Average Nutrient Percent.")

  Name of this report in my software program: _____

- A report that provides your average energy expenditure information for the days you tracked your activities. (In the manual, this report will be called "Average Energy Expenditure.")

  Name of this report in my software program: _____

Analyzing Diet and Activity Manually on the Web

If you do not have a computer software program available to analyze your diet and activity habits, you can analyze them manually or use a Web-based program. You can find the nutrient composition of foods on the Web at the United States Department of Agriculture Web site: http://www.nal.usda.gov/fnic/foodcomp/search.

You can complete Part IIB: MyPyramid Diet Analysis manually or by using the Web-based assessment available at http://www.mypyramid.gov using MyPyramid Tracker. This online assessment can analyze your food intake and your physical activity and compare them to the Dietary Guidelines and the MyPyramid recommendations for food groups, nutrients, and energy balance.

Another online dietary assessment option is the "Interactive Healthy Eating Index." You can find this assessment at the MyPyramid Web site within the MyPyramid Tracker section. It is also available at the USDA Web site: http://www.usda.gov/cnpp/. This online assessment tool allows you to score your dietary quality for 1 day or up to 20 days. The Healthy Eating Index measures how well your diet complies with the recommendations of the Dietary Guidelines for Americans and MyPyramid.

You access your activity level manually using the directions found in Assessment 8.2. Rather than simply calculate for one day, determine your energy expenditure manually for as many days as you need to complete. Make additional copies of this page to complete this manually.

Source: B. Mayfield. (2006). *Personal Nutrition Profile,* 2nd ed. Sudbury, MA: Jones and Bartlett, 1–10.

Name: _____ Course Number: _____

Section: _____ Date: _____

Part A: MyPyramid Analysis of Diet

The first assessment of your diet will be to compare your food intake to the recommended amounts from each of the food groups on MyPyramid. This will give you a good idea of how well your diet meets the nutrition principles of variety, balance, and moderation. MyPyramid emphasizes three key messages:

- Make smart choices from every food group.
- Find your balance between food and physical activity.
- Get the most nutrition out of your calories.

MyPyramid is pictured on the next page. This graphic represents a personalized approach to healthy eating and physical activity. To view a color graphic, go to the MyPyramid Web site: http://www.mypyramid.gov. Variety is represented by the six color bands, which represent the five food groups of the Pyramid and oils. Moderation is represented by the narrowing of each food group band from bottom to top, with the wider base for foods with little or no solid fats or added sugars to be selected more often than the foods with more fat and sugar found at the top. Proportionality is shown by the different widths of the food group bands. The widths suggest how much food a person should choose from each group. Activity is represented by the person climbing the steps. The slogan "Steps to a Healthier You" encourages gradual improvement by taking small steps to improve your diet and lifestyle each day.

To begin your assessment, go to the MyPyramid Web site: http://www.mypyramid.gov. You will be asked to enter your age, sex, and activity level. To determine your activity level, refer to your activity records and add up the minutes of moderate, vigorous, or strenuous activity you do daily that is in addition to your normal daily routine. You will have three options of activity levels: less than 30 minutes, 30–60 minutes, and more than 60 minutes. Entering this data will result in your own "MyPyramid Plan" listing the recommended amounts of food from each food group, amount of fats and oils, and amount of discretionary calories. This is based on one of 12 calorie patterns, as in the table on page 85. Print out a PDF version of your results and/or fill in your recommendations on page 89.

To compare your daily food intake with your recommended intake in each food group, you can use the online MyPyramid Tracker or do it manually using the table and instructions on page 87. To do the analysis online, click on "MyPyramid Tracker." Follow the online instructions to assess your food intake. You can also use this tool to assess your physical activity. You will be asked to log in after you have selected one of the two assessment options. A more personalized assessment will be made with this tool accounting for not only your age and gender, but also your height and weight.

Enter your food intake for each 24-hour period you recorded using the corresponding date in your personal profile. When you have entered all foods, you can analyze your food intake for each day by clicking "save and analyze." You can compare your intake to the 2005 Dietary Guidelines, your MyPyramid recommendations, your recommended nutrient intakes, and also your healthy eating history. This site also computes your Healthy Eating Index score. Fill in page 88 for MyPyramid Diet Analysis.

To do this analysis manually, turn to page 87.

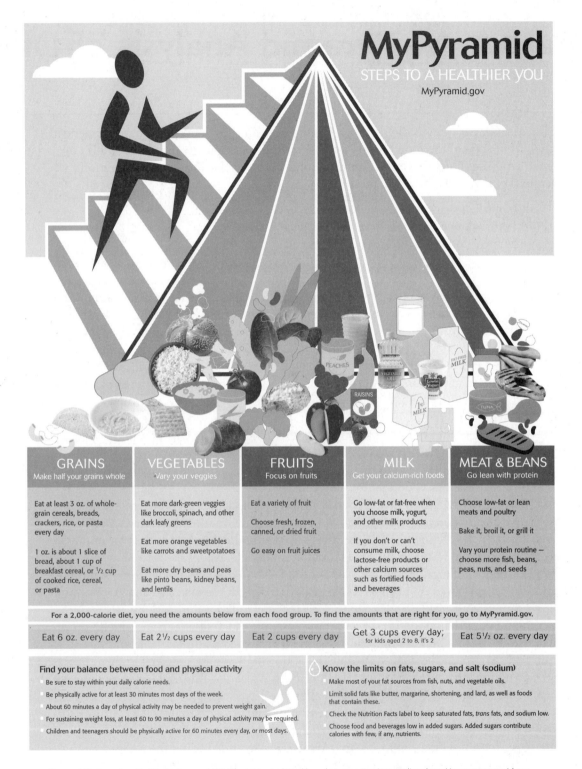

Source: U.S. Department of Agriculture and U.S. Department of Health and Human Services. Online: http://www.mypyramid.gov.

MyPyramid Food Intake Patterns

The following table lists suggested amounts of food to consume from the five basic food groups and oils to meet recommended nutrition intakes at 12 different calorie levels for adults and children over the age of 2. There are no food intake pattern calorie levels for adults below 1600 calories. For young adults ages 19–30, the calorie range for females is 2000–2400, and the calorie range for males is 2400–3000, depending on activity level. Nutrient and energy contributions from each group are calculated according to the nutrient-dense forms of foods in each group (e.g., lean meats and fat-free milk). The table also shows the discretionary calorie allowance that can be accommodated within each calorie level.

Daily Amount of Food from Each Group												
Calorie Level	1000	1200	1400	1600	1800	2000	2200	2400	2600	2800	3000	3200
Fruits[1] (in cups/day)	1	1	1.5	1.5	1.5	2	2	2	2	2.5	2.5	2.5
Vegetables[2] (in cups/day)	1	1.5	1.5	2	2.5	2.5	3	3	3.5	3.5	4	4
Grains[3] (in ounce-equivalents/day)	3	4	5	5	6	6	7	8	9	10	10	10
Meat and Beans[4] (in ounce-equivalents/day)	2	3	4	5	5	5.5	6	6.5	6.5	7	7	7
Milk[5] (in cups/day)	2	2	2	3	3	3	3	3	3	3	3	3
Oils[6] (in teaspoons/day)	3	4	4	5	5	6	6	7	8	8	10	11
Discretionary Calorie Allowance[7] (total remaining calories)	165	171	171	132	195	267	290	362	410	426	512	648

Refer to the chart on pages 86–87 for types and amounts of foods in each food group that count as the equivalent of a cup or ounce-equivalent.

1. The Fruit Group includes all fresh, frozen, canned, and dried fruits and fruit juices.

2. The Vegetable Group includes all fresh, frozen, canned, and dried vegetables and vegetable juices. Five vegetable subgroups are recommended each week:

Dark green vegetables	(3 cups/week)
Orange vegetables	(2–2.5 cups/week)
Legumes	(3–3.5 cups/week)
Starchy vegetables	(3–9 cups/week)
Other vegetables	(6.5–10 cups/week)

For your recommended amounts from each subgroup, refer to the "MyPyramid Plan" you calculated at http://www.mypyramid.gov.

3. The Grains Group includes all foods made from wheat, rice, oats, cornmeal, and barley, such as bread, pasta, oatmeal, breakfast cereals, tortillas, and grits. At least half of all grains consumed should be whole grains.

4. The Meat and Beans Group includes meat, poultry, fish, eggs, nuts, nut butters, legumes (cooked dry beans), tofu, and seeds.

5. The Milk Group includes all fluid milk products and foods made from milk, such as yogurt and cheese.

6. Oils include fats from many different plants and from fish that are liquid at room temperature, such as canola, corn, olive, soybean, and sunflower. Some foods are naturally high in oils, like nuts, olives, some fish, and avocados. Foods that are mainly oil include mayonnaise, certain salad dressings, and soft margarine.

7. The discretionary calorie allowance is the amount of calories remaining after accounting for the calories needed for all food groups (using only foods that are fat-free or low-fat and with no added sugars) and oils. It allows you to select higher fat and sugar options from the food groups, as well as "extras." For more information go to "Inside the Pyramid" and then click on "Discretionary Calories" at the MyPyramid Web site.

Food Group Equivalents

Grains (1 ounce-equivalents)
Make at least half your grains whole-grain choices.

1 regular slice bread	½ small bagel	½ hamburger bun
1 small 6" tortilla	½ cup cooked pasta	1 small pita
½ cup cooked rice	1 cup flaked cereal	1¼ cups puffed cereal
½ cup cooked oatmeal	1 4½" pancake	½ medium Danish or donut
(1 instant packet)	1 waffle	½ large croissant
½ English muffin	4–6 crackers	3 graham crackers
1 8" breadstick	1 plain, small roll	1 1¼" × 2½" corn bread
1 ounce pretzels	3 cups popcorn	2 taco shells
1 muffin (2½" diameter)	1 biscuit (2" diameter)	¼ cup prepared stuffing

Vegetables (1 cup equivalents)
Emphasize variety and color.

1 cup raw or cooked vegetables
2 cups raw leafy vegetables
1 2½–3" diameter baked potato
1 cup cooked dry beans or peas*
1 cup ½" tofu cubes*
1 cup (8 oz) 100% vegetable juice
20 French fries
1 large ear of corn

Fruits (1 cup equivalents)
Emphasize variety and color.

1 (2½–3" diameter) piece fresh fruit
1 cup berries or cut-up fruit
1 cup canned fruit or applesauce
1 cup (8 oz) 100% fruit juice
1 large banana (8–9" long)
1 medium grapefruit (4" diameter)
2 large plums (or 3 medium)
½ cup dried fruit

Milk, Yogurt, and Cheese (1 cup equivalents)
Select fat-free and low-fat dairy foods.

1 cup (8 oz) milk, plain or flavored
1 cup (8 oz) plain or fruit-flavored yogurt
1½ ounce natural cheese
⅓ cup shredded cheese
2 ounces processed (American) cheese

½ cup ricotta cheese
2 cups cottage cheese
1 cup frozen yogurt
1½ cups ice cream
1 cup pudding made with milk

Meat and Beans (1 ounce-equivalents)
Select lean cuts of meat, poultry without skin.

1 ounce cooked beef, poultry, pork, or fish
Items that each count as 1 ounce of meat:

1 egg or ¼ cup fat-free egg alternative	1 Tbsp peanut butter
¼ cup cooked dry beans or peas*	½ ounce nuts or seeds
½ cup bean soup	¼ cup tofu (~2 ounces)*
2 Tbsp hummus	½ veggie burger (soy) patty

Oils
Select fats derived from plant sources and/or fish.

Contains 3 tsp oil	*Contains 2½ tsp oil*	*Contains 2 tsp oil*
1 Tbsp oil (such as canola or olive)	1 Tbsp soft margarine	2 Tbsp oil-based salad dressing
½ medium avocado	1 Tbsp mayonnaise	16 large olives
1 ounce sunflower seeds	2 Tbsp creamy salad dressing	1 ounce nuts (peanuts, cashews, almonds)
1 Tbsp peanut butter		

*Starchy beans, peas, and tofu can be counted toward either vegetables or meats.

Manual MyPyramid Diet Analysis

Use the table on page 88 (making copies as needed) to list the foods and beverages you consumed on each of the days you kept diet records. Use one table for each of the different days. Write your name and the date of each diet record in the spaces provided.

List the food or beverage in the first column, and the amount eaten in equivalents of cups and ounces in the column corresponding to the appropriate food group. Refer to the Food Group Equivalents chart on pages 86 and 87. Use decimals to indicate partial servings. Be sure to list all food groups represented in combination foods. Note that some foods can be counted as either vegetables or meat/beans.

In the summary table on page 89, calculate the average amount of food consumed in each group (total amount divided by the number of days). If the amount in any food group fell below the recommended amount, write the amount indicating the shortage in the row labeled "shortage." (For example, if you should have had 6 ounce-equivalents in the grain group and only had 4, write 2 in the space to indicate your shortage.) If the amount you consumed in any food group exceeded the amount recommended, write the number indicating the surplus in the row labeled "Surplus." (For example, if you should have had 5.5 ounce-equivalents in the meat group and you had 8, write 2.5 in the space to indicate your surplus.)

Fats and oils are recommended in teaspoons per day. See the Food Group Equivalents chart to assist you in computing teaspoons of oil from added fats in your diet.

Discretionary calories can include both calories from foods in the food groups or from sweets and alcohol. Use the discretionary calorie column to list calories from sweets and alcohol, which do not fit within any of the food group columns. Use food labels or lists such as the food composition tables in your textbook to find the amount of calories. Keep in mind that "sugar" on a food label includes both natural and added sugars. Sweetened beverages generally have 100 calories per 8-ounce cup. A serving of alcohol is considered 12 ounces of beer, 1.5 ounces of liquor, or 4–5 ounces of wine or cocktails. These range in calories from about 80 calories for 4 ounces of wine, to 100 calories for 1.5 ounces of liquor, to 150 calories for a 12-ounce beer.

MyPyramid Diet Analysis

Day: _____

Name: _____ Date: _____

My Intake: Food or Beverage	Amount Eaten in Food Groups (ounce or cup equivalents)						
	Grains (oz-equiv)	Vegetable (cups)	Fruit (cups)	Milk (cups)	Meat (oz-equiv)	Oils (tsp)	Discretionary Calories

Name: _____

Total Daily Amount Eaten in MyPyramid Food Groups							
	Grains (oz-equiv)	Vegetable (cups)	Fruit (cups)	Milk (cups)	Meat (oz-equiv)	Oils (tsp)	Discretionary Calories
Day One							
Day Two							
Day Three							
Day Four							
Day Five							
Day Six							
Day Seven							
Average (Total ÷ # of Days)							
Recommended (Refer to your MyPyramid Plan)							
Shortage							
Surplus							

Target Behavior: Meet my recommended intake within energy needs by adopting a balanced eating plan. Using MyPyramid Plan, I will select a variety of foods and eat the recommended amount in each food group.

Food group(s) in which I met the recommended amount of food most days:

_____

Food group(s) in which I ate *less than* the recommended amount of food most days:

_____

Food group(s) in which I ate *more than* the recommended amount of food most days:

_____

Name: _____ Course Number: _____

Section: _____ Date: _____

Part B: Macronutrient Assessment

Sources of Calories

a. Fill in the following table to compare *your* average daily intake of macronutrients to the Dietary Reference Intakes set forth by the Food and Nutrition Board, Institute of Medicine, National Academy of Sciences (2002). (See the reports titled "Average Nutrient Intake" and "Average Nutrient Percent.")

	Average Daily Intake (grams)	Average kcal from Macronutrient	Average Total Calories*	Share of Total Calories (%)	Recommended Share of Calories (%)
Carbohydrates	____ × 4 =	____ ÷	____ =	____	45–65%
Total Fat	____ × 9 =	____ ÷	____ =	____	20–35%
Protein	____ × 4 =	____ ÷	____ =	____	10–35%

*The "average total calories" should be the *same* number in each calculation, equal to the average number of calories you eat in one day.

b. Assess how well you met this recommendation for distribution of calories, allowing for no more than a small contribution of calories (less than 10%) from alcohol. Do you need to eat more of one macronutrient and less of another to fit within the acceptable ranges?

Carbohydrate, Fiber, and Sugar Intake

a. Did you consume at least the minimum recommended amount**
   of carbohydrate (130 grams) needed to produce enough glucose
   for the brain to function?   ____ yes ____ no

b. On average, how many grams of dietary fiber did you eat each day?   ____ g

c. Did you eat the recommended** grams of fiber on average
   each day? (25 grams for women, 38 grams for men)   ____ yes ____ no

d. List the foods you consumed with the *most* dietary fiber *per serving*. (See the reports titled "Nutrient Composition of Foods" or the food composition tables in your textbook.)

**Dietary Reference Intakes for macronutrients set forth by the National Academy of Sciences Institute of Medicine, 2002.

Food	Fiber (g)	Food	Fiber (g)
_____	_____	_____	_____
_____	_____	_____	_____
_____	_____	_____	_____
_____	_____	_____	_____

e. If you did *not* meet the recommended amount of fiber, what are three foods that you would be willing to eat regularly that contain 3 or more grams of fiber per serving?

Food	Fiber (g)
_____	_____
_____	_____
_____	_____

f. What foods and beverages did you consume that provided carbohydrates in the form of added sugar in your diet (e.g., candy, cookies and cakes, soft drinks)? List the items that contributed the highest amounts of sugar to your diet and how many calories were provided by each food. If the information is available, list how many grams of added sugar are in each food and calculate how many calories are provided by added sugars. (See the reports titled "Nutrient Composition of Foods" or the nutrient composition of foods on the Web at http://www.ars.usda.gov/ba/bhnrc/ndl.)

Food	Calories from Food	Grams of Added Sugars		Calories from Sugar
_____	_____	_____	× 4 kcal/g =	_____
_____	_____	_____	× 4 kcal/g =	_____
_____	_____	_____	× 4 kcal/g =	_____
_____	_____	_____	× 4 kcal/g =	_____
_____	_____	_____	× 4 kcal/g =	_____

g. How many total calories did these foods provide in your diet? _____ calories (This amount is the *total* calories in these foods, not just the calories from sugar.)

h. How much does that average per day (divide by number of days)? _____ calories/day

i. Is your average intake of calories from these foods higher than your "discretionary calorie allowance" (see MyPyramid Diet Analysis, page 89)? _____ yes _____ no

j. What percentage of your total calories comes from added sugars? Total calories from sugar: _____ ÷ Total calories consumed × 100 = _____ % kcal from added sugars

---

- The 2005 Dietary Guidelines recommend you "Choose and prepare foods and beverages with little added sugars or caloric sweeteners."
- The USDA Food Guide and MyPyramid consider added sugars a portion of the "discretionary calorie allowance."
- A National Academy of Sciences Report (2002) (available at http://books.nap.edu/openbook.php?record_id=104908page-R1) recommends that no more than 25 percent of total calories come from added sugars.

---

k. Would you consider your intake of foods with added sugars moderate or high?

_____ moderate _____ high

l. If your intake is high (i.e., you checked "no" for item i), what could you eat or drink *less* of?

_____

Fat and Cholesterol Intake

a. Did 20–35 percent of your *total* calories come from fat? _____ yes _____ no

b. Figure your average percentage of total calories from saturated fat:

1. Average daily intake of saturated fat from "Average Nutrient Intake" report = _____ g

2. Multiply by 9 kcal/g = _____ kcal from saturated fat.

3. Divide by your total average calories and multiply by 100 to get _____ percent of calories from saturated fat.

c. Did you meet the recommendation of less than 10 percent of total calories?* _____ yes _____ no

d. According to your daily "Nutrient Composition of Foods" reports, list the top five sources of fat and saturated fat in your diet:

Sources of Fat	(g)	Sources of Saturated Fat	(g)

e. According to your daily "Nutrient Composition of Foods" reports or food labels, what foods did you eat that were sources of trans fats? What alternates could you select to limit your intake of trans fats?

Sources of Trans Fat	Alternate Food Sources
_____	_____
_____	_____
_____	_____

f. According to your "Average Nutrient Intake" report, what is your average daily intake of cholesterol: _____ mg

g. Did you meet the recommendation to consume no more than 300 mg of cholesterol per day?* _____ yes _____ no

h. According to your daily "Nutrient Composition of Foods" report, what foods contribute the *most* cholesterol to your diet?

Sources of Cholesterol	(mg)	Sources of Cholesterol	(mg)
_____	_____	_____	_____
_____	_____	_____	_____
_____	_____	_____	_____
_____	_____	_____	_____

*The American Heart Association and the National Cholesterol Education Program recommend that less than 10 percent of total calories come from saturated fats and less than 300 mg of cholesterol be consumed daily.

Protein Intake

a. Was your average percentage of calories from protein 10–35 percent? _____ yes _____ no

b. Your personal Recommended Dietary Allowance (RDA) for protein is based on your healthy weight. Calculate your RDA for protein by following these steps:

1. Convert your *healthy weight** in pounds to kilograms:
   Divide healthy weight in pounds by 2.2 = _____ kg

   If you are not sure if you are within your healthy weight range, look at the BMI chart found in your textbook (or the NHLBI Web site). A healthy weight for your height is one with a BMI value between 19 and 25. If your weight is above or below this range, select the weight in the healthy range closest to your current weight and convert it to kilograms.

2. Multiply your *healthy weight* in kilograms by 0.8 g protein/kg weight to determine your RDA for protein:
   _____ kg body weight × 0.8 g/kg = _____ g protein

c. Did your average protein intake meet or exceed your RDA for protein? _____ yes _____ no

d. Using your "Nutrient Composition of Foods" reports, list the top five sources of animal protein (this includes milk and eggs) and plant protein in your diet, and indicate the grams of protein per portion of food you ate:

Animal Sources of Protein	**(g)**	**Plant Sources of Protein**	**(g)**
_____	_____	_____	_____
_____	_____	_____	_____
_____	_____	_____	_____
_____	_____	_____	_____
_____	_____	_____	_____
Total	_____	**Total**	_____

e. Did you eat more protein (in total grams) from animal sources or plant sources?

_____

f. Consider the benefits of increasing the sources of plant protein in your diet. If you ate more protein from animal sources than from plant sources, list four plant-based foods you could eat more regularly that provide *at least* 5 grams of protein per serving.

_____   _____

_____   _____

g. Using the assessments you completed, indicate how often you meet the target behaviors listed below and on page 96.

Macronutrient Target Behaviors	**Always/ Usually**	**Some- times**	**Rarely/ Never**
• Consume at least 130 grams carbohydrate per day	_____	_____	_____
• Consume at least 25 or 38 grams of total fiber per day (25 g for females, 38 g for males)	_____	_____	_____
• Moderate intake of added sugars	_____	_____	_____
• Consume no more than 35 percent of total calories from fats	_____	_____	_____
• Consume less than 10 percent of total calories from saturated fats	_____	_____	_____

Macronutrient Target Behaviors	Always/ Usually	Some- times	Rarely/ Never
• Consume less than 300 mg cholesterol	——	——	——
• Consume little or no trans fats	——	——	——
• Meet RDA for protein	——	——	——
• Obtain a significant contribution of protein from plant sources	——	——	——

Describe below how well your diet meets the recommendations for macronutrient intake. Compose a short paragraph (five to six sentences) that describes the overall contribution of calories from carbohydrate, fat, and protein in your diet; whether your intake of fiber is adequate; whether your intakes of sugar, fat, saturated fat, trans fat, and cholesterol are healthy or excessive; and whether you consume adequate protein and types of protein in your diet.

_____

_____

_____

_____

Source: B. Mayfield. (2006). *Personal Nutrition Profile*, 2nd ed. Sudbury, MA: Jones & Bartlett, 18–29.

Name: ——————————————————— Course Number: ———————————

Section: ——————————————————— Date: ———————————————

Part A: Lifestyle Behavior Readiness Assessment

The following 12 descriptions of healthy lifestyle behaviors are based on the Dietary Guidelines for Americans (2005), U.S. Department of Health and Human Services (HHS), and U.S. Department of Agriculture (USDA). The Dietary Guidelines include 41 key recommendations, 23 for the general public and 18 for special populations, grouped into 9 general topic areas. The report is available at http://www.healthierus.gov/dietaryguidelines.

Read each of the following lifestyle behavior descriptions (titled "Dietary Guidelines Key Messages"), then select the statement from the list that best expresses your intentions or current practice. Circle the letter(s) that signifies your intent.

Codes for Stages of Readiness for Behavioral Change

PC = Precontemplation — Description of target behavior doesn't match my current behavior patterns, and I don't intend to change them to be more like it in the next 6 months.

C = Contemplation — Description of target behavior doesn't match my current behavior patterns, but I do intend to change them to be more like it in the next 6 months.

P = Preparation — Description of target behavior doesn't match my current behavior patterns, but I am motivated and confident that I can change them to be more like it in the next 30 days.

A = Action — Description of target behavior is similar to my current behavior patterns, but I've only been practicing this behavior for less than 6 months.

M = Maintenance — Description of target behavior is similar to my current behavior patterns, and I've been doing this for 6 months or longer.

Dietary Guidelines Key Messages	*Stages of Change*
1. Balance Food and Physical Activity To maintain body weight in a healthy range, balance calories from foods and beverages with calories expended.	PC C P A M
2. Be Physically Active Each Day Engage in physical activity totaling at least 30 minutes most days of the week to reduce risk of disease, at least 60 minutes most days to prevent weight gain, or at least 60–90 minutes to sustain weight loss. Reduce sedentary activities.	PC C P A M

Dietary Guidelines Key Messages   Stages of Change

3. Achieve Physical Fitness
   Engage in cardiovascular conditioning, stretching
   exercises for flexibility, and resistance exercises
   or calisthenics for muscle strength and endurance.

PC	C	P	A	M

4. Make Your Calories Count
   Consume a variety of nutrient-dense foods and
   beverages within and among the basic food groups.

PC	C	P	A	M

5. Choose a Variety of Fruits and Vegetables
   Eat a colorful variety of fruits and vegetables daily.
   Select vegetables from all five subgroups several
   times a week.

PC	C	P	A	M

6. Make Half Your Grains Whole
   Eat at least 3 ounces of whole-grain cereals,
   bread, crackers, rice, or pasta every day.

PC	C	P	A	M

7. Get Your Calcium-Rich Foods
   Get at least 3 cups of low-fat or fat-free milk,
   or an equivalent amount of low-fat yogurt and/or
   low-fat cheese every day.

PC	C	P	A	M

8. Choose Fats Wisely
   Eat less saturated fat, trans fat, and cholesterol.
   Use more monounsaturated and polyunsaturated
   fats and oils. Choose lean meats, fish, poultry,
   legumes, and low-fat dairy products more often.

PC	C	P	A	M

9. Choose Carbohydrates Wisely
   Choose fiber-rich fruits, vegetables, and whole
   grains often. Choose and prepare foods and
   beverages with little added sugars or caloric
   sweeteners.

PC	C	P	A	M

10. Choose and Prepare Foods with Little Salt
   Consume less than 2300 mg (approximately
   1 teaspoon of salt) of sodium per day.

PC	C	P	A	M

**11. If You Drink Alcoholic Beverages,
   Do So Sensibly and in Moderation**
   Limit intake to no more than one drink per day for
   women, and no more than two drinks per day for men.

PC	C	P	A	M

12. Keep Food Safe to Eat
   Clean hands, food contact surfaces, and fruits
   and vegetables. Avoid cross-contamination of
   foods. Store and serve food at safe temperatures.

PC	C	P	A	M

Lifestyle Behavior Readiness Assessment

Name: _____ Course Number: _____

Section: _____ Date: _____

Part B: MyPyramid Goal Setting

MyPyramid Behavioral Readiness and Goal Setting

You will select one food group that you would benefit from modifying your intake to more consistently meet the recommendations of your personal MyPyramid plan. If your assessment determined that your consumption of all food groups generally meets the recommended intake, select one group to concentrate on for *maintaining* the recommended intake (select the food group that challenges you most). For example, if you consume the recommended daily amount of vegetables, determine whether your weekly intake of the five vegetable subgroups matches the recommended amounts. Assess your "stage of change" for adopting the desired behavior of consuming the recommended daily intake in the food group you selected.

Food group I plan to work on: _____
(If you're not sure which food group to select, choose one with a *shortage* in preference to one with a *surplus*. Generally, meeting a goal of consuming *more* is easier than eating *less*, and it often results in eating less in those food groups in which you have a surplus.)

Current behavior: _____
                  (This is your current average intake from the food group listed above.)

Target behavior: **Meet my recommended intake within energy needs by adopting a balanced eating plan. Using MyPyramid Plan, I will select a variety of foods and eat the recommended amount in each food group.**

To consistently eat _____ from the _____ group daily.
         (amount in cups or ounce-equivalents)   (fill in food group listed above)

Stage of readiness for change: _____
                  (Select the stage from the following list that best describes your intention to change.)

Codes for Stages of Readiness for Behavioral Change

PC = Precontemplation   Description of target behavior doesn't match my current behavior patterns, and I don't intend to change them to be more like it in the next 6 months.

C = Contemplation   Description of target behavior doesn't match my current behavior patterns, but I do intend to change them to be more like it in the next 6 months.

P	**= Preparation**	Description of target behavior doesn't match my current behavior patterns, but I am motivated and confident that I can change them to be more like it in the next 30 days.
A	**= Action**	Description of target behavior is similar to my current behavior patterns, but I've only been practicing this behavior for less than 6 months.
M	**= Maintenance**	Description of target behavior is similar to my current behavior patterns, and I've been doing this for 6 months or longer.

Select the goal-setting worksheet (Assessment 2.2) that corresponds to your stage of change. Make a photocopy of it before filling in the worksheet. Complete the entire worksheet.

_____

_____

_____

_____

Source: B. Mayfield. (2006). *Personal Nutrition Profile,* 2nd ed. Sudbury, MA: Jones & Bartlett, 54–56.

MyPyramid Goal Setting

Name: —————————————————————— Course Number: ——————————————

Section: —————————————————————— Date: ——————————————————

Chapter 7: Critical Thinking Questions

Optimal Nutrition for an Active Lifestyle

1. Like Terri, you might sometimes rely on dietary suplements. What supplements are you currently taking or have you taken? For each supplement, list natural foods that you could eat that provide you the same nutritional value as the supplement.

2. Identify three barriers you face in trying to follow the *Dietary Guidelines for Americans*. For each barrier, identify a strategy and timeline to overcome it.

3. You are one of 12 students at your university who is asked to assist the dietetics staff in developing healthy, nutritious, and appealing meals for college students. Using your nutrition knowledge, develop a well-balanced menu for breakfast, lunch, and dinner.

4. Go to a local health food store (often you can find one in a shopping mall). Walk through the store and look at the products and their health claims. Find two products, identify the claims made, and note any scientific research that supports the claim. Would you, based on the information provided, use this product? Why or why not?

Critical Thinking Questions

Name: ——————————————————— Course Number: ———————————————

Section: ——————————————————— Date: ———————————————————

Body Weight Assessment

Body Weight Assessment

a. Assess your current weight status based not only on your height and weight, and therefore on your body mass index (BMI), but also by looking at your weight history and weight distribution. Keep in mind that weight is only *one* indicator of your overall health. Your health history, personal health profile, diet, eating habits, activity, fitness, stress, and emotional health are *all* important to your health and well-being.

Height in inches: ——————————— ÷ 39.3 = height in meters: ———————————

Weight in pounds: ——————————— ÷ 2.2 = weight in kilograms: ———————————

Calculate your BMI:

Weight (kg)/height (m)² = ——————————— ÷ (———————————)² = BMI of ———————————
(weight in kg)   (height in m²)

Compare this BMI calculated using your height and weight to the BMI values in your textbook. They should be the same.

b. What is the health risk associated with your BMI? (Refer to the following table.)

Risk Level	BMI (Men and Women)
Lowest risk	19–24.9
Increased risk	25–29.9
Moderate risk	30–34.9
High risk	35–39.9
Very high risk	40 or higher
Risk also increases with BMIs of less than 19.	

c. Do you have any preexisting conditions or risk factors that could increase your risk (e.g., cardiovascular disease risk, elevated blood lipids, diabetes)? If so, what are they?

——

Weight History

a. Describe your weight during the following periods in your life.

Early elementary:	_____ underweight	_____ average weight	_____ overweight
Upper elementary:	_____ underweight	_____ average weight	_____ overweight
Middle school:	_____ underweight	_____ average weight	_____ overweight
High school:	_____ underweight	_____ average weight	_____ overweight

b. What is the *most* and *least* you have weighed as an adult (since graduating from high school)?   most: _____ age: _____
least: _____ age: _____

c. Describe how much your weight fluctuates.   lowest: _____ highest: _____

Weight Distribution

Where you carry your weight affects your risk for a variety of health problems. Upper body weight (the "apple" shape) increases your risk. Lower body weight (the "pear" shape) lowers your risk, but is more difficult to lose.

a. Determine how your weight is distributed by using your waist circumference. Measure your waistline by placing a tape measure around your waist (at the top of your hip bone). Do not hold your breath or pull in your stomach muscles while taking the measurement, and relax while standing straight with your feet together.

My waist circumference: _____

> Men: Your risk increases if your waist circumference exceeds 40 inches.
> Women: Your risk increases if your waist circumference exceeds 35 inches.

b. Are you at increased risk due to waist circumference?   _____ yes   _____ no

Healthy Weight

a. Considering your current weight, your weight history, the stability of your weight, the risk associated with your BMI, and your weight distribution, what do you consider a healthy weight for you?

Current weight: _____   **Healthy weight:** _____

b. If your healthy weight is different from your current weight, what is a reasonable and safe weight change goal?

> A reasonable weight loss goal does not exceed 10 percent of your body weight.
> A safe rate of weight loss or gain is no more than 0.5–2 pounds per week.

Weight change goal: _____ Maintain weight in current range

_____ Lose _____ pounds by _____

_____ Gain _____ pounds by _____

Source: B. Mayfield. (2006). *Personal Nutrition Profile*, 2nd ed. Sudbury, MA: Jones & Bartlett, 40–41.

Name: _____   Course Number: _____

Section: _____   Date: _____

Energy Balance

a. Using your "Daily Nutrient Intake" and "Daily Energy Expenditure" reports, compare your daily *intake* of energy with your daily *expenditure* of energy (fill in the appropriate number of weekdays and weekend days):

Weekday 1:	Intake was	_____ kcal	Expenditure was	_____ kcal
Weekday 2:	Intake was	_____ kcal	Expenditure was	_____ kcal
Weekday 3:	Intake was	_____ kcal	Expenditure was	_____ kcal
Weekday 4:	Intake was	_____ kcal	Expenditure was	_____ kcal
Weekday 5:	Intake was	_____ kcal	Expenditure was	_____ kcal
Weekend Day 1:	Intake was	_____ kcal	Expenditure was	_____ kcal
Weekend Day 2:	Intake was	_____ kcal	Expenditure was	_____ kcal

b. Compare your *average* energy intake with your *average* energy expenditure. Divide your total intake values and your total expenditure values listed above by the number of days.

Average intake of calories per day:	_____ **kcal/day**
Average expenditure of calories per day:	_____ **kcal/day**

c. What is the average difference?   _____ kcal/day

What is the direction of the difference?
_____ Intake sometimes greater, expenditure sometimes greater; balances out over time.
_____ Intake more often greater than expenditure.
_____ Expenditure more often greater than intake.

d. Is this difference a true reflection of your tendency to gain, lose, or maintain weight?

_____ yes   _____ no

If not, explain why:
(Possible explanations include underreporting intake, overreporting expenditure, database inaccuracy, and days not typical. *Ideally, your recorded days will be typical.*)

_____

_____

_____

_____

e. Does your energy intake and/or energy expenditure differ between weekdays and weekend days?

_____ yes _____ no

If so, how do they differ and which factors contribute to the difference?

_____

_____

Understanding Energy Expenditure

a. Calculate your energy expenditure manually for one day of your choice to better understand how your body burns calories for various activities as well as for simply staying alive.

Date selected: _____

1. Calculate your energy use for *basal metabolism*:
This is the energy your body needs just to stay alive (basic bodily functions) 24 hours a day.

Female: _____ (kg weight; see page 103) × 0.9 kcal/kg/h × 24 hours = _____ **kcal**
(1)

Male: _____ (kg weight; see page 103) × 1.0 kcal/kg/h × 24 hours = _____ **kcal**
(1)

2. Calculate your energy use for the *thermic effect of food* (TEF):
This is the energy your body needs for digestion, absorption, and nutrient utilization. It varies between individuals. This exercise uses 10%.

Caloric intake _____ kcal × 0.10 = _____ **kcal**
(2)

3. Calculate your energy use for *physical activity*:
This energy use is over and above the calories being burned to maintain vital body functions and food utilization; it is the energy expended solely for the purpose of supporting your level of activity. Using your activity record for the day you selected, add up the total number of minutes spent at each of the following activity levels. Multiply this number by your weight in kilograms and the number of kilocalories expended per minute per kilogram. The result is your calories used or expended.

Activity Level	Time Spent (minutes)	Weight (kg)	Kcal/min/kg	Calories Expended
Sedentary			0.01	
Light			0.02	
Moderate			0.03	
Vigorous			0.06	
Strenuous			0.10	
Total Calories Expended for Physical Activity				

(3)

4. Calculate your *total energy expenditure*:

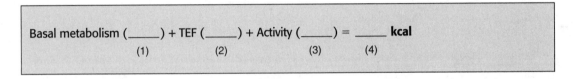

Basal metabolism (_____) + TEF (_____) + Activity (_____) = _____ **kcal**

            (1)   (2)   (3)   (4)

Source: B. Mayfield. (2006). *Personal Nutrition Profile,* 2nd ed. Sudbury, MA: Jones & Bartlett, 42–43.

Name: _____ Course Number: _____

Section: _____ Date: _____

Estimating and Changing Your Resting Metabolic Rate

Estimating Your Resting Metabolic Rate

Directions: A simple calculation can provide a rough estimate of your resting metabolic rate (RMR). However, remember that your RMR can vary greatly from this estimate due to your fitness level, sex, size, body composition, pregnancy status, age, whether you have eaten recently, environmental temperature, drugs and medications, hormone secretion status, and health status.

To Calculate RMR

1. Measure your body weight (BW) in kilograms. _____

2. Measure your height (HT) in centimeters. _____

3. Record your age in years. _____

4. Insert those items into the appropriate equation below and perform the calculation. The result is your RMR in kcal.

Men RMR $= 66.473 + 13.751$ (BW) $+ 5.0033$ (HT) $- 6.755$ (age)
Women RMR $= 655.0955 + 9.463$ (BW) $+ 1.8496$ (HT) $- 4.6756$ (age)

This calculation is valid for adults 20–40 years of age.

Changing Your Resting Metabolic Rate

Directions: The most effective way to increase your resting metabolic rate (RMR) is through resistance training. By performing strength training exercises, you add muscle mass to your body. Muscle tissue is more active tissue than is adipose tissue, so your metabolic rate will increase. In addition, larger people tend to have higher RMRs than smaller people.

To See How a 10-lb Addition of Muscle Mass Will Impact Your RMR

1. Measure your body weight (BW) in kilograms (kg). _____

2. Add 4.5 kg to that number (BW+). _____

3. Measure your height (HT) in centimeters. _____

4. Record your age in years. _____

5. Insert those items into the appropriate equation that follows and perform the calculation.

The result is your new RMR. In fact, adding 10 lbs of muscle will potentially bring about an even higher RMR.

Men RMR = 66.473 + 13.751 (BW+) + 5.0033 (HT) − 6.755 (age)
Women RMR = 655.0955 + 9.463 (BW+) + 1.8496 (HT) − 4.6756 (age)

Source: J.A. Harris & F.G. Benedict. (1919). *A Biometric Study of Basal Metabolism in Man* (Pub. No. 279). Washington, DC: Carnegie Institute. Reprinted with permission.

Name: _____   Course Number: _____

Section: _____   Date: _____

How Do You Feel About Your Body?

	Quite Satisfied	Somewhat Satisfied	Somewhat Dissatisfied	Very Dissatisfied
Hair	_____	_____	_____	_____
Arms	_____	_____	_____	_____
Hands	_____	_____	_____	_____
Feet	_____	_____	_____	_____
Waist	_____	_____	_____	_____
Buttocks	_____	_____	_____	_____
Hips	_____	_____	_____	_____
Legs and ankles	_____	_____	_____	_____
Thighs	_____	_____	_____	_____
Chest or breasts	_____	_____	_____	_____
Posture	_____	_____	_____	_____
General attractiveness	_____	_____	_____	_____

1. Which of your thoughts and actions enhance your body image?

_____

_____

2. Which of your thoughts and actions are detrimental to your body image?

_____

_____

3. What societal forces (expectations of friends and parents, advertising, celebrities and professional athletes, etc.) influence your body image most strongly?

_____

_____

4. How susceptible are you to media images of "ideal" body proportions for members of your sex?

_____

_____

5. What could you do to become more satisfied with your body image?

_____

_____

Source: G. Edlin & E. Golanty. (2007). *For Your Health: A Study Guide and Self-Assessment Workbook.* Sudbury, MA: Jones & Bartlett, 77.

Chapter 8: Critical Thinking Questions

Achieving and Maintaining a Healthy Weight

1. From the vignette, how would you assess Denise's preoccupation with her weight? What factors influence her concerns about her weight? Do you believe she has an unhealthy obsession with her weight?

2. On your campus, identify and briefly describe the resources available for students regarding healthy weight management and eating disorders.

3. Your housemate, Linda, goes on a new fad diet that was recently reported by a respected national morning TV show. Linda reports that this new diet will allow her to lose 10 pounds by Saturday (6 days from now). Explain to Linda why this fad diet will not work, and if she were to lose the 10 pounds in 6 days, what would likely happen.

4. As a residence hall assistant (RA) you have been asked by your floor to talk about obesity and how as college freshmen they can manage their weight sensibly. In your talk, discuss healthy weight, overweight and obesity, body mass index, and the importance of good nutrition and physical activity.

Name: _____ Course Number: _____

Section: _____ Date: _____

Are You Consuming Enough Calcium?

According to statistics from the U.S. Department of Agriculture, only 1 in 10 girls and 1 in 3 boys ages 12 to 19 in the United States get the Recommended Dietary Allowance (RDA) of calcium, placing them at serious risk for osteoporosis and other bone diseases. Because nearly 90 percent of adult bone mass is established by the end of this age range, the nation's young adults stand in the midst of a calcium deficiency crisis. The daily calcium requirements by age and sex from Table 9.1 in your textbook are reprinted here.

Age and Sex	Adequate Daily Intake of Calcium (mg)
Infants, male or female, 0–6 months	210
Infants, male or female, 7–12 months	270
Children, male or female, 1–3 years	500
Children, male or female, 4–8 years	800
Males and females, 9–18 years	1300
Males and females,* 19–50	1000
Males and females,† 51 years and older	1200
Pregnant or lactating female, 14–18 years	1300
Pregnant or lactating female, 19–50 years	1000

*If you are female and in menopause, you should increase your calcium intake to 1200 mg.
†Some clinicians recommend 1500 mg of calcium per day for postmenopausal women.

Source: I.M. Alexander. (2006). 100 Questions and Answers About Osteoporosis and Osteopenia. Sudbury, MA: Jones & Bartlett, 95.

Record your calcium intake from the foods you eat for a week (see Table 9.2 in your textbook for a list of selected food sources of calcium). Are you obtaining enough calcium in your diet from food? If not, what foods could you include in your diet to increase your daily calcium intake?

_____

_____

Have you thought about taking a dietary calcium supplement? Why or why not?

_____

_____

Name: _____ Course Number: _____

Section: _____ Date: _____

Are You Performing Enough Weight-Bearing Exercise?

Physical activity plays an important role in improving bone health, specifically because bone mass is responsive to mechanical loads (stress) placed on the skeleton. Bone becomes stronger and denser when you place demands on it. Examples of weight-bearing exercises for adults from Table 9.5 in your textbook are reprinted here.

Weight-Bearing, High-Impact, and/or Resistance Activities

Stair climbing

Hiking

Dancing

Jogging

Downhill and cross-country skiing

Aerobic dancing

Volleyball

Basketball

Gymnastics

Weight lifting or resistance training

Soccer

Jumping rope

Weight-Bearing, Low-Impact Activities

Walking

Treadmill walking

Cross-country ski machines

Stair-step machines

Rowing machines

Water aerobics

Deep-water walking

Low-impact aerobics

Minimal Weight-Bearing, Nonimpact Activities

Lap swimming

Indoor cycling

Stretching or flexibility exercises
(avoid forward-bending exercises)

Yoga

Pilates

Source: National Osteoporosis Foundation. (2003). *Boning Up on Osteoporosis: A Guide to Prevention and Treatment.* Washington, DC: Author.

Which of the weight-bearing exercises listed in the table do you regularly perform on a daily or weekly basis?

_____

_____

_____

_____

Based on the scientific information provided in Chapter 9 on the role of physical activity and bone health, do you feel that your current physical activity program related to weight-bearing and resistance exercises is adequate for your skeletal health? Why or why not?

_____

_____

_____

_____

_____

_____

_____

_____

_____

_____

_____

_____

_____

_____

_____

_____

_____

_____

_____

_____

_____

_____

_____

_____

Are You Performing Enough Weight-Bearing Exercise?

Name: _____ Course Number: _____

Section: _____ Date: _____

My Osteoporosis Risk

Directions

1. Go to the online assessment tool "Your Disease Risk: The Source on Prevention" at http://www.yourdiseaserisk.wustl.edu. Here, you can find out your risk of developing osteoporosis in the United States and get personalized tips for preventing osteoporosis.

2. Click the What's your osteoporosis risk? link, and then click Questionnaire.

3. Is your risk low, average, or high? _____

4. Click the What makes up my risk? button and list the factors that raise your risk and the factors that lower your risk.

Factors that raise my risk of osteoporosis: _____

Factors that lower my risk of osteoporosis: _____

Name: _____ Course Number: _____

Section: _____ Date: _____

Chapter 9: Critical Thinking Questions

Achieving Optimal Bone Health

1. Like Julie, many people do not understand that both physical inactivity and low calcium intake are key factors in the development of osteoporosis. You have been asked by a local ninth-grade health teacher to explain to her students the importance of physical activity and nutrition in preventing osteoporosis (a condition that is the last thing on most ninth-graders' minds). In 250 words or less, explain their importance.

2. Review the factors that affect osteoporosis (genetic, hormonal, nutritional, and lifestyle). Review your family history to determine if you are at risk of osteoporosis. Then select two other factors and, based on your current behaviors, decide what behaviors you could change that would assist in preventing osteoporosis. List them.

3. "Physical activity and nutrition are key elements in achieving optimal bone density during the first 20 to 30 years of life and maintaining bone density throughout life." Provide information that supports that statement.

_____

_____

_____

_____

_____

_____

_____

_____

_____

_____

_____

_____

_____

_____

_____

Critical Thinking Questions

Name: ———————————————————————— Course Number: ————————————

Section: ———————————————————————— Date: ————————————————

K6 Serious Psychological Distress Assessment

Answer the following questions by checking the box that best applies.

During the past 30 days, how often did you feel . . .	All of the time 4	Most of the time 3	Some of the time 2	A little of the time 1	None of the time 0
So sad that nothing could cheer you up?					
Nervous?					
Restless or fidgety?					
Hopeless?					
That everything was an effort?					
Worthless?					
Total					

Scoring: To score the K6, add the points for each of the questions together. Scores can range from 0 to 24. A threshold of 13 or more points indicates a high degree of distress and possibility of serious mental illness.

Source: National Center for Health Statistics. (2007). Serious psychological distress. Online: http://www.cdc.gov/nchs/data/ad/ad382.pdf.

Name: _____ Course Number: _____

Section: _____ Date: _____

Time Management

Activity 1: Ranking Tasks

Step 1

Write down all the things you need to get done today with no regard to order of importance.

1. _____   6. _____
2. _____   7. _____
3. _____   8. _____
4. _____   9. _____
5. _____   10. _____

Step 2

In column A, list all the things that must get done as soon as possible. In column C, list all the things you would like to do, but that are not essential. In column B, put everything else.

A	B	C
_____	_____	_____
_____	_____	_____
_____	_____	_____
_____	_____	_____

Activity 2: Scheduling

After completing Activity 1: Ranking Tasks and determining what needs to get done, complete your schedule.

7:00 a.m. _____

7:30 a.m. _____

8:00 a.m. _____

8:30 a.m. _____

9:00 a.m. _____

9:30 a.m. _____

10:00 a.m. _____

10:30 a.m. _____

11:00 a.m. _____

11:30 a.m. _____

12:00 p.m. _____

12:30 p.m. _____

1:00 p.m. _____

1:30 p.m. _____

2:00 p.m. _____

2:30 p.m. _____

3:00 p.m. _____

3:30 p.m. _____

4:00 p.m. _____

4:30 p.m. _____

5:00 p.m. _____

5:30 p.m. _____

6:00 p.m. _____

6:30 p.m. _____

7:00 p.m. _____

7:30 p.m. _____

8:00 p.m. _____

8:30 p.m. _____

9:00 p.m. _____

9:30 p.m. _____

10:00 p.m. _____

10:30 p.m. _____

11:00 p.m. _____

10.3

Name: _____ Course Number: _____

Section: _____ Date: _____

Relaxation Techniques

Activity 1: Progressive Muscle Relaxation

Progressive muscle relaxation involves three steps that can help you actually feel the difference between tension and relaxation. First, tense a muscle and notice how it feels. Second, release the tension and pay attention to that feeling. Third, rest, concentrating on the difference between the two sensations. Perform these steps while either sitting or lying down, preferably in a quiet, soothing environment.

It takes only about 10 minutes to exercise all the major muscle groups. There are several sequences. You can start with the hand muscles, progressing to others; begin at the top, moving from head to toe; or reverse the direction, going from bottom to top as explained in the following section.

Procedure

This sequence of exercises progresses from the feet to the head and takes about 10 minutes. Its effectiveness comes from alternately tensing and relaxing each muscle group. Hold tense, then relax for about 5 seconds each.

1. Curl toes tightly. Hold, Relax, Rest
2. Flex the feet. Hold, Relax, Rest
3. Tighten the calves. Hold, Relax, Rest
4. Tense the thighs. Hold, Relax, Rest
5. Tighten the buttocks. Hold, Relax, Rest
6. Tighten the lower back. Hold, Relax, Rest
7. Tighten the abdomen. Hold, Relax, Rest
8. Tense the upper chest. Hold, Relax, Rest
9. Tense the upper back muscles. Hold, Relax, Rest
10. Clench the fists. Hold, Relax, Rest
11. Extend the fingers and flex the wrists. Hold, Relax, Rest
12. Tighten the forearms. Hold, Relax, Rest
13. Tighten the upper arms. Hold, Relax, Rest
14. Lift the shoulders gently toward the ears. Hold, Relax, Rest

15. Wrinkle the forehead. Hold, Relax, Rest

16. Squeeze your eyes shut. Hold, Relax, Rest

17. Drop your chin, letting your mouth open wide. Hold, Relax, Rest

18. Lift the shoulders gently and then pull them down as if you had weights in the hands. Hold, Relax, Rest

Activity 2: The Relaxation Response

The relaxation response tends to banish inner stress and exert a calming, healing influence. It not only helps preserve emotional balance in everyday life, but it also enhances therapy for a host of illnesses, especially high blood pressure. Herbert Benson developed the following simple, practical procedure for eliciting the relaxation response.

Procedure

1. Select a focus word or brief phrase that has deep meaning for you.

2. Take a comfortable sitting position in a quiet environment.

3. Close your eyes and consciously relax your muscles.

4. Breathe slowly and naturally through your nose while silently repeating your focus word or phrase each time you inhale.

5. Keep your attitude passive; disregard thoughts that drift in.

6. Continue for 10 to 20 minutes once or twice a day.

You can pick almost any focus word or phrase, such as the word "one." Some meditators find it helpful to focus on the breath—in, out, in, out—rather than on a word or phrase. Others prefer to focus on an object, such as a candle flame. If you want to time your session, peek at a watch or clock occasionally, but don't set a jarring alarm. Getting to your feet immediately after a session can make you feel slightly dizzy, so sit quietly for a few moments first with your eyes closed. The technique works best on an empty stomach, either before a meal or about 2 hours after eating. Avoid those times when you are obviously tired unless you want to fall asleep. Although you will feel refreshed after the first session, it may take a month or more to get noticeable results, such as lower blood pressure.

After trying the two relaxation techniques in Activities 1 and 2 (progressive muscle relaxation; relaxation response) several times each, which do you prefer?

_____

Why?

_____

_____

Use your preferred relaxation technique daily over a 2-week period of time. Identify for each day your location, approximate length of time taken, and your feelings when finished.

Your preferred method: _____

	Date:	Date:	Date:	Date:	Date:	Date:	Date:
Location							
Length							
Feelings: calm, relaxed, etc.							

	Date:	Date:	Date:	Date:	Date:	Date:	Date:
Location							
Length							
Feelings: calm, relaxed, etc.							

Name: _____ Course Number: _____

Section: _____ Date: _____

Creative Problem Solving

Activity 1: Scenarios

Directions

Choose one of the following problems. This activity can provide good practice for the times when you will need to apply these skills to real life.

Problem 1: Paul is called into his supervisor's office and told that the company must lay off some employees. Paul will be laid off in 2 months. He is married and has two small children. He has a mortgage payment on his home and a car payment each month.

Problem 2: You are upset after having an argument with your junior high school–aged son about the trouble he is getting into at school.

Problem 3: Maria has four final exams and only 2 days left to study for them. She is anxious because she doesn't think she will have enough time to study for the exams.

Which of the problems did you choose? _____

1. Define the problem.

   _____

   _____

   _____

2. List the facts.

   _____

   _____

3. List possible solutions (at least four).

   a. _____

   _____

   b. _____

   _____

   c. _____

   _____

   d. _____

   _____

4. Analyze and evaluate the possible solutions.

_____

_____

_____

5. Select one solution to implement.

_____

_____

_____

6. Evaluate the results (for this assignment, give ways you would evaluate).

_____

_____

_____

Activity 2: Problem-Solving Steps

Write a problem that was or is stressing you. Go through the problem-solving steps. Write the problem:

_____

_____

_____

1. Define the problem.

_____

_____

_____

2. List the facts.

_____

_____

_____

3. List possible solutions (at least four).

a. _____

_____

_____

b. _____

_____

_____

c. _____

_____

_____

d. _____

_____

_____

4. Analyze and evaluate the possible solutions.

_____

_____

_____

5. Select one solution to implement.

_____

_____

_____

6. Evaluate the results (for this assignment give ways you would evaluate).

_____

_____

_____

Name: _____ Course Number: _____

Section: _____ Date: _____

Chapter 10: Critical Thinking Questions

Mental Health and Coping with Stress

1. Jackson was able to determine that exercising helped relieve the speech anxiety he was having. Review Figure 10.5 and Figure 10.6 in the textbook. Are you experiencing any of the harmful stress symptoms listed? If so, do you think stress is the cause? If yes, what are the specific stressors? What physical activities might you do to help relieve these stressors?

2. Review your list of life stress sources. Next to each source, list whether you would use environmental engineering, mind engineering, or physical engineering to manage the stressor. Would more than one strategy be useful? Do you see physical activity helping to manage the stress in your life? Why or why not?

3. Stressors can be a result of situations present on your campus or in your campus community. Community stressors may be problems such as crime, pollution, lack of recreation facilities, and overcrowded classrooms or residence halls. Identify what you consider to be a major stressor in your campus community. How would you go about changing this stressor?

_____

_____

_____

_____

_____

_____

_____

_____

_____

_____

_____

_____

_____

Critical Thinking Questions

Name: _____ Course Number: _____

Section: _____ Date: _____

Do You Have a Drinking Problem?

This questionnaire is designed to help you determine whether you have a problem with alcohol. Answer each question yes or no and record your choice in the left hand column.

Yes	No		
____	____	**1.**	Do you believe you are a normal drinker?
____	____	**2.**	Have you ever awakened after drinking the night before and found that you could not remember some part of the evening?
____	____	**3.**	Does your wife, husband, a parent, or other near relative ever worry or complain about your drinking?
____	____	**4.**	Can you stop drinking without a struggle after one or two drinks?
____	____	**5.**	Do you ever feel bad about your drinking?
____	____	**6.**	Do friends or relatives think you are a normal drinker?
____	____	**7.**	Do you ever try to limit your drinking to certain times of the day or to certain places?
____	____	**8.**	Are you always able to stop drinking when you want to?
____	____	**9.**	Have you ever attended a meeting of Alcoholics Anonymous?
____	____	**10.**	Have you gotten into fights when drinking?
____	____	**11.**	Has drinking ever created problems between you and your wife, husband, boyfriend, girlfriend, a parent, or other near relative?
____	____	**12.**	Has your wife, husband, boyfriend, girlfriend, a parent, or other near relative ever gone to anyone for help about your drinking?
____	____	**13.**	Have you ever lost friends because of drinking?
____	____	**14.**	Have you ever gotten into trouble at work because of drinking?
____	____	**15.**	Have you ever lost a job because of drinking?
____	____	**16.**	Have you ever neglected your obligations, your family, or your work for two or more days in a row because you were drinking?
____	____	**17.**	Do you drink before noon fairly often?
____	____	**18.**	Have you ever been told you have liver trouble? Cirrhosis?
____	____	**19.**	After heavy drinking have you ever had delirium tremens (DTs) or severe shaking?
____	____	**20.**	After heavy drinking have you ever heard voices or seen things that weren't really there?
____	____	**21.**	Have you ever gone to anyone for help about your drinking?
____	____	**22.**	Have you ever been in a hospital because of drinking?
____	____	**23.**	Have you ever been a patient in a psychiatric hospital or in a psychiatric ward of a general hospital?

_____ _____ **24.** Have you ever been in a hospital to be "dried out" (detoxified) because of drinking?

_____ _____ **25.** Have you ever been in jail, even for a few hours, because of drunk behavior?

Scoring

Item keying for alcoholic responses are 1. N; 2. Y; 3. Y; 4. N; 5. Y; 6. N; 7. Y; 8. N; 9–25, Y. To score, add one point for each alcoholic response.
The total score is the number of alcoholic responses.

Number of Alcoholic Responses	Interpretation
0–2	No problem with alcohol
3–5	Early warning signs that drinking is becoming problematic
6 or more	Problem drinker/alcoholic

If you think you have a drinking problem, seek professional help.

Source: G. Edlin, E. Golanty, & K. McCormack Brown. (1999). _Health and Wellness,_ 6th ed. Sudbury, MA: Jones & Bartlett, 401.

Do You Have a Drinking Problem?

Name: _____ Course Number: _____

Section: _____ Date: _____

Why Do You Smoke?

Here are some statements made by people to describe what they get out of smoking cigarettes. How often do you feel this way when smoking? Circle one number for each statement.

Important: Answer every question.

	Always	Frequently	Occasionally	Seldom	Never
A. I smoke cigarettes to keep myself from slowing down.	5	4	3	2	1
B. Handling a cigarette is part of the enjoyment of smoking it.	5	4	3	2	1
C. Smoking cigarettes is pleasant and relaxing.	5	4	3	2	1
D. I light up a cigarette when I feel angry about something.	5	4	3	2	1
E. When I have run out of cigarettes I find it almost unbearable until I can get them.	5	4	3	2	1
F. I smoke cigarettes automatically without even being aware of it.	5	4	3	2	1
G. I smoke cigarettes to stimulate me, to perk myself up.	5	4	3	2	1
H. Part of the enjoyment of smoking a cigarette comes from the steps I take to light up.	5	4	3	2	1
I. I find cigarettes pleasurable.	5	4	3	2	1
J. When I feel uncomfortable or upset about something, I light up a cigarette.	5	4	3	2	1
K. I am very much aware of the fact when I am not smoking a cigarette.	5	4	3	2	1
L. I light up a cigarette without realizing I still have one burning in the ashtray.	5	4	3	2	1
M. I smoke cigarettes to give me a lift.	5	4	3	2	1
N. When I smoke a cigarette, part of the enjoyment is watching the smoke as I exhale it.	5	4	3	2	1

	Always	Frequently	Occasionally	Seldom	Never
0. I want a cigarette most when I am comfortable and relaxed.	5	4	3	2	1
P. When I feel blue, or want to take my mind off cares and worries, I smoke cigarettes.	5	4	3	2	1
Q. I get a real gnawing hunger for a cigarette when I haven't smoked for a while.	5	4	3	2	1
R. I've found a cigarette in my mouth and I didn't remember putting it there.	5	4	3	2	1

How to Score

1. Enter the numbers you have circled in the following spaces, putting the number you have circled to Question A over line A, to Question B over line B, and so forth.

2. Add the three scores on each line to get your totals. For example, the sum of your scores over lines A, G, and M gives you your score on Stimulation, lines B, H, and N give the score on Handling, and so on.

Totals

A	+	G	+	M	=	Stimulation
B	+	H	+	N	=	Handling
C	+	I	+	O	=	Pleasurable relaxation
D	+	J	+	P	=	Crutch; tension reduction
E	+	K	+	Q	=	Craving: psychological addiction
F	+	L	+	R	=	Habit

Scores of 11 or above indicate that this factor is an important source of satisfaction for the smoker. Scores of 7 or less are low and probably indicate that this factor does not apply to you. Scores in between are marginal.

Source: Smoker's Self-Testing Kit developed by Daniel Horn, PhD. Originally published by National Clearinghouse for Smoking and Health, Department of Health, Education, and Welfare.

Name: _____ Course Number: _____

Section: _____ Date: _____

The Drugs You Take

Keep a list of all the nonessential drugs that you ingest for a week. Be sure to include coffee, tea, and cola drinks (which contain caffeine); alcohol; nicotine; and pain relievers. After the first week, look at your list. Are you surprised by how many of these nonessential drugs you use? Now, keep the list for another week, but eliminate just one of the nonessential drugs that you ingest and make notes about how you feel.

Week 1	Sun	Mon	Tue	Wed	Thu	Fri	Sat

Caffeine

(How many cups of coffee or 12-oz servings of cola drinks per day?) _____

Alcohol

(How many 12-oz beers, glasses of wine, or mixed drinks per day?) _____

Nicotine

(How many cigarettes, cigars, pipes, or dips of snuff or chewing tobacco per day?) _____

Pain relievers

(How many tablets per day?) _____

Other: _____

Other: _____

Week 2	Sun	Mon	Tue	Wed	Thu	Fri	Sat

Caffeine

(How many cups of coffee or 12-oz servings of cola drinks per day?) _____

Alcohol

(How many 12-oz beers, glasses of wine, or mixed drinks per day?) _____

Nicotine

(How many cigarettes, cigars, pipes, or dips of snuff or chewing tobacco per day?) _____

Pain relievers

(How many tablets per day?) _____

Other: _____

Other: _____

Source: G. Edlin & E. Golanty. (2007). *For Your Health: A Study Guide and Self-Assessment Workbook.* Sudbury, MA: Jones & Bartlett, 135.

© 2011 Jones & Bartlett Learning

Name: _____ Course Number: _____

Section: _____ Date: _____

Chapter 11: Critical Thinking Questions

Making Informed Decisions About Drug Use

1. "I really don't like the taste of liquor that much, but after the first couple of shots, it doesn't taste all that bad. I know I shouldn't drink and I always have a hangover the next day but, hey, college is stressful and how else can I deal with the stress of getting the grades to keep my scholarship and making my parents happy?" What's your opinion of this person's attitude? Explain why you agree or disagree. If you disagree, how do you think this person can deal with the stress of getting good grades?

2. College campuses often accept money from companies that sell alcoholic beverages—to support athletic events, for example. By allowing these companies to advertise at campus events, the university makes considerable money to enhance the campus environment and provide quality education. What is your campus's policy on allowing alcohol companies to advertise or sponsor events on campus? Do you agree or disagree with this policy?

3. Purchase a popular magazine and count the number of cigarette ads in the issue. In reviewing each of the ads, respond to the following questions:

    a. Who is the ad targeting (young people, older adults, women)?

    b. How is the ad appealing to the target audience (fun, sex)?

    c. What does the ad seem to promise if you smoke their brand of cigarette?

    _____

    _____

    _____

    _____

    _____

    _____

    _____

    _____

    _____

    _____

    _____

    _____

Critical Thinking Questions

Name: _____ Course Number: _____

Section: _____ Date: _____

Skeptical Buyer Exercise

Locate an advertisement selling an exercise product (such as an infomercial or magazine advertisement) and answer the following questions.

1. What is the name of the product?

_____

2. What is the purported purpose of the product?

_____

3. What marketing strategies are being used to persuade you to purchase the product? See Table 12.2 in the textbook.

_____

_____

_____

4. In your opinion, is the product worth what the company is selling it for?

_____

_____

_____

5. What portions of the marketing strategy are suspect?

_____

_____

_____

6. Would you buy the product? Why or why not?

_____

_____

_____

Name: _____ Course Number: _____

Section: _____ Date: _____

Health Club Evaluation

Visit a local health/fitness club and answer the following questions.

1. What population is the club designed to serve?

_____

2. What are the best aspects of the club?

_____

_____

_____

3. What are the worst aspects of the club?

_____

_____

_____

4. How much are dues?

_____

5. What qualifications do the exercise instructors have?

_____

_____

_____

6. What services are offered in the club?

_____

_____

_____

7. Would you join the club? Why or why not?

_____

_____

_____

Chapter 12: Critical Thinking Questions

Health Consumerism

1. Like Janet, you are constantly bombarded with advertisements about a diet pill or drink that will guarantee losing X pounds per week. These advertisements are often displayed on college and university campuses. As you walk to class, take a look around to see if you notice any of these advertisements. Record what you see. Also, review the most recent issue of your college or university newspaper. Are there any ads for fad diets or pills? If so, who are they targeting?

2. In a popular magazine, find an advertisement that you believe might be misleading or fraudulent. Determine which of the advertising approaches are used to convince readers to purchase the product. What argument would you present to counter the advertising claims?

3. Speculate about why people often fall victim to common physical activity and health misconceptions, frauds, or fallacies.

4. As a critical health consumer, where would you suggest peers go to find valid information on physical activity and health? Give three sources and explain how you determined they were valid.

_____

_____

_____

_____

_____

_____

_____

_____

_____

_____

_____

_____

_____

Critical Thinking Questions

Name: _____ Course Number: _____

Section: _____ Date: _____

Thinking About Your "Relationship Portfolio"

There are several things to consider in a relationship portfolio, including the type of each relationship, the number of people in it, the time spent in those relationships, and the quality of each relationship. Much like a financial investment portfolio for retirement, diversifying (or expanding) and reflecting on your relationship portfolio is important.

Complete the following relationship portfolio chart based on the following types of relationships you read about in Chapter 13: acquaintances/casual friends, work/school relationships, internet-based relationships, family, best friends, and romantic partners.

Types of Relationships	Acquaintances/ Casual Friends	Work/ School	Internet-Based	Family	Best Friends	Romantic Partners
Number of relationships						
Time (per day) spent in relationships						
Quality of relationships+						

+Importance scale: 1 = unimportant; 2 = somewhat important; 3 = important; 4 = very important

Reflection Activity

Each type of relationship can play a valuable and different role in our lives. Take some time to reflect on your relationship portfolio by answering the following questions.

1. Are you weighted too heavily in one relationship category?

_____

_____

2. Are you missing some important relationships that you wish you had?

_____

_____

_____

3. Compare the amount of time you spend in each type of relationship with the importance of the relationship type to you. Do you want to make any adjustments? For example, do you want to spend more time in some of your relationships, or do you want more relationships in a particular category?

_____

_____

_____

4. What adjustments might you consider making to the quantity, quality, or amount of time spent in your relationships?

_____

_____

_____

Small Group Activity

Consider how many close or best friends you would like. How much time do you want to spend with your best friends? Discuss the following questions about close friendships in your small groups.

1. How can I develop close friendships and ways to meet new people? Share why you think close relationships are important.

_____

_____

2. What circumstances prompt you to call on your close relationships (e.g., best friends, family, romantic partners)?

_____

_____

3. For what types of things do you seek support? For example, who do you call when you do not do well on a test? Who do you call for support if you have an argument with another friend or a family member?

_____

_____

4. What types of things do you feel comfortable sharing with your acquaintances/casual friends?

_____

_____

Name: _____ Course Number: _____

Section: _____ Date: _____

How Much Do You Know About Healthy Relationships?

The answers are given on the next page.

1. A healthy way to show that you are listening to someone is to:

   a. Say: "It seems like you're saying you would like me to call you if I'm going to be late".

   b. Look the person in the eye when he or she is speaking.

   c. Wait until the other person has finished speaking before you say something.

   d. All of the above

2. If you want to talk with your friend about something private, which is the best way to do this?

   a. Demand to speak with your friend right away when he or she is in a big group of people.

   b. Find your friend when he or she is alone so that you can talk privately together.

   c. Don't say anything because it's better to hold your feelings inside.

   d. Stop talking to your friend until he or she asks what's wrong.

3. A healthy way to show your hurt feelings is by saying which of the following statements?

   a. "You make me mad when you do that."

   b. "I hate you when you don't do what I want."

   c. "I feel upset when you do that."

   d. "You should know what I'm feeling."

4. If you and a good friend are having an argument that you can't seem to work out, what should you do?

   a. Tell your friend that you won't talk to her or him until she or he says you're right.

   b. Talk behind her or his back with all your other friends.

   c. Ask a trusted adult for help.

   d. Storm out of the room and slam the door behind you.

5. If you and a good friend are going through a tough time, it might help you to do which of the following?

    a. Ignore your friend and spend all your time with other people.

    b. Blame all the problems on yourself.

    c. Stop listening to what the other person has to say.

    d. Remember that you care about each other and try to listen extra hard to each other.

6. What is one way to know if friends really care about you?

    a. They like that you help them with their math homework all the time.

    b. They are happy for you when you do well.

    c. They don't say they are sorry if they hurt your feelings because friends don't have to apologize.

    d. They like to give you advice so that you do things the way that they do them.

7. Which one of these will not help you make new friends?

    a. Introducing yourself and remembering people's names

    b. Not joining a new club because you are not sure you will like it

    c. Getting involved in after-school activities

    d. Being sensitive to other people's feelings

8. What should you do if your friends pressure you to drink?

    a. Be strong and say, "I don't want to."

    b. Spend time with other friends who don't pressure you, and also make new friends.

    c. Suggest other things that you and your friends can do for fun.

    d. All of the above

Answers to How Much Do You Know About Healthy Relationships?

1. D. Having good listening skills is very important for all relationships. One way to show someone that you are listening is to repeat what was said so you do not misunderstand him or her. Looking at a person when he or she is talking to you and not interrupting are two additional ways to show you are listening.

2. B. The best idea is to speak with your friend alone. You may want to quietly pull your friend aside and arrange a later time to speak in private. In a healthy relationship, it is important to share your feelings. If you are having trouble talking to your friend about something, think about talking to a trusted adult.

3. C. A good way to show your feelings is by using "I statements." Voicing your feelings this way helps you to be direct, honest, and positive instead of blaming others. In order to have healthy relationships, you need to tell people how you are feeling. No one can read your mind, even if they are really close to you! Try using statements such as, "I feel mad/sad/upset/etc. when you don't listen to me."

4. C. Sometimes you may find that an argument is getting nowhere and you and your friend may need help from a trusted adult. Talk with someone who won't take sides so they can listen to what you both have to say. You may find that sitting down together with an adult will help you to organize your thoughts so you can work things out.

5. D. Even in healthy relationships, people disagree and argue. Difficult times may pass if you are able to talk about your feelings with one another. Healthy relationships take time and energy.

6. B. Your true friends want you to be happy and are happy for you when things go your way. If someone only likes you because you help them, doesn't say he or she is sorry for hurting your feelings, or always wants you to do things their way, this person is not a true friend.

7. B. Here are some great ways to help you make new friends: Introduce yourself and try to remember people's names, get involved in after-school activities, and be sensitive to other people's feelings. New friends will appreciate all of these things!

8. D. All of these options are good choices to help you handle a pressure-filled situation involving alcohol.

Source: Online: http://www.girlshealth.gov/relationships/quizzes/quiz.relknow.cfm.

Name: _____ Course Number: _____

Section: _____ Date: _____

How Much Do You Know About Ways to Deal with Conflict?

The answers are given on the next page.

1. If you're feeling angry, what should you do?

   a. Stomp around the room but say nothing.

   b. Slam the door, hard.

   c. Ignore your friend at school.

   d. Carefully tell your friend what you are feeling.

2. By not dealing with conflict in a healthy way, what could happen?

   a. You could loose a good friend.

   b. You could not be treated unfairly at work or school.

   c. You could not get something you want or need.

   d. You might feel like you can never make things better.

   e. All of the above

3. True or False: Counting to 10 before speaking if you're feeling angry is a healthy way of dealing with conflict.

   a. True

   b. False

4. Which statement can help people stay open and honest when there is a conflict?

   a. "You only think about yourself!"

   b. "I feel upset when you don't ask me what I want to do."

   c. "You don't care about me!"

   d. "You will never be happy with my homework!"

5. How can you stay safe from violence?

   a. Choose your friends carefully.

   b. Report any weapons to a trusted adult.

   c. Practice "safety in numbers."

   d. All of the above

   e. None of the above

6. True or False: Staying calm during a disagreement with your parents can help show them that you are growing up.

a. True

b. False

7. True or False: You should never compromise when you are mad at someone.

a. True

b. False

Answers to How Much Do You Know About Ways to Deal with Conflict?

1. D. If you're feeling angry, you should carefully tell your friend what you are feeling.

2. E. By not dealing with conflict in a healthy way, you could lose a good friend, be treated unfairly at work or school, not get something you want or need, and/or feel like you can never make things better.

3. A. Counting to 10 before speaking if you're feeling angry is a healthy way of dealing with conflict.

4. B. A great way of letting someone know how you feel is to use an "I statement" and to stat your true feelings, such as "I feel upset when you don't ask me what I want to do."

5. D. To stay safe from violence choose your friends carefully, report any weapons to a trusted adult, and practice "safety in numbers."

6. A. Staying calm during a disagreement with your parents can help show them that you are growing up.

7. B. You should compromise when you are mad at someone.

Source: Online: http://www.girlshealth.gov/relationships/quizzes/quiz.conflict.cfm.

After completing Activity 13.3, ask yourself if there is room for growth in your relationships or in the way you deal with conflict. Answer these questions, and then discuss them in small groups.

1. For you, what makes it hard to address conflict directly for you?

2. Are there times or when certain people with whom you find it harder or easier to address conflict?

3. What goals do you have for improving the way you deal with conflict?

Name: _____ Course Number: _____

Section: _____ Date: _____

Am I in an Abusive Relationship?

Does Your Partner . . .

Embarrass you with put-downs?	Yes	No
Look at you or act in ways that scare you?	Yes	No
Control what you do, who you see or talk to, or where you go?	Yes	No
Stop you from seeing your friends or family members?	Yes	No
Take your money or Social Security check, make you ask for money or refuse to give you money?	Yes	No
Make all of the decisions?	Yes	No
Tell you that you're a bad parent or threaten to take away or hurt your children?	Yes	No
Prevent you from working or attending school?	Yes	No
Act like the abuse is no big deal, it's your fault, or even deny doing it?	Yes	No
Destroy your property or threaten to kill your pets?	Yes	No
Intimidate you with guns, knives, or other weapons?	Yes	No
Shove you, slap you, choke you, or hit you?	Yes	No
Force you to try and drop charges?	Yes	No
Threaten to commit suicide?	Yes	No
Threaten to kill you?	Yes	No

If you answered yes to even one of these questions, you may be in an abusive relationship.

For support and more information, please call the National Domestic Violence Hotline at 1-800-799-SAFE (7233) or TTY 1-800-787-3224.

Be Safe. Computer use can be monitored and is impossible to completely clear. If you are afraid your Internet and/or computer usage might be monitored, please use a safer computer, call your local hotline, and/or call the National Domestic Violence Hotline at 1-800-799-SAFE (7233) or TTY 1-800-787-3224.

Source: National Domestic Violence Hotline. Online: http://www.ndvh.org/is-this-abuse/am-i-being-abused-2.

Chapter 13: Critical Thinking Questions

Developing Healthy Social and Intimate Relationships

1. Read the following scenario and identify several communication problems. How could Bob and Sandy have handled this situation using healthy communication skills?

   Bob: Well, Sandy, you know that this weekend is the big reunion of all my fraternity brothers, and I'd like you to join me in celebrating our 100-year anniversary!

   Sandy: Now you ask! I've already told my theater group that we would join them for their weekend outing.

   Bob: Great, you didn't even ask me, you just went ahead and made plans for me this weekend!

   Sandy: Ask you? You have been so busy lately with work and school, I haven't even had a chance to talk to you let alone ask you if you wanted to spend the weekend with me and the theater group.

   Bob: Oh great, now it is my fault that I've been working so hard and trying to get good grades. Go ahead, blame it on me!

   Sandy: Okay! It's your fault we never spend any time together. I'm sick of this! What will it be, your fraternity brothers or me?

   Bob: Well, now I'm having to choose between you and my fraternity brothers. That's easy! My fraternity brothers any day—at least they understand how hard it is to work and go to school!

2. "An intimate relationship may be sexual, but a sexual relationship is not necessarily an intimate one." Discuss the difference(s) between an intimate relationship and a sexual relationship.

3. Identify 10 terms that are gender-biased. Example: fireman.

4. Identify five television shows that have characters in stereotypical male or female roles. Identify the characters and briefly explain the roles they play.

5. Do you and/or your romantic partner wish to increase your level of communication? If so, what steps might you take to do so?

6. Identify at least three ways that healthy relationships can improve your physical health. How are your relationships contributing to your physical health?

7. Discuss the positives and negatives of having online friendships.

8. What are some of the risks of text messaging something important?

9. Identify some movies or television shows in which there was a conflict between two close friends or romantic partners. Discuss what they may have been able to do differently to deal with the conflict and improve their communication.

_____

_____

_____

_____

_____

_____

_____

_____

_____

_____

_____

_____

_____

_____

_____

_____

_____

_____

_____

_____

_____

_____

_____

_____

_____

Name: _____ Course Number: _____

Section: _____ Date: _____

Check Your Cholesterol and Heart Disease IQ

Directions: Are you cholesterol smart? Test your knowledge about high blood cholesterol with the following statements. Mark each true or false. The answers are given on the next page.

	True	False
1. High blood cholesterol is one of the risk factors for heart disease that you can do something about.	____	____
2. To lower your blood cholesterol level you must stop eating meat altogether.	____	____
3. Any blood cholesterol level below 240 mg/dL is desirable for adults.	____	____
4. Fish oil supplements are recommended to lower blood cholesterol.	____	____
5. To lower your blood cholesterol level you should eat less saturated fat, total fat, and cholesterol, and lose weight if you are overweight.	____	____
6. Saturated fats raise your blood cholesterol level more than anything else in your diet.	____	____
7. All vegetable oils help lower blood cholesterol levels.	____	____
8. Lowering blood cholesterol levels can help people who have already had a heart attack.	____	____
9. All children need to have their blood cholesterol levels checked.	____	____
10. Women don't need to worry about high blood cholesterol and heart disease.	____	____
11. Reading food labels can help you eat the heart-healthy way.	____	____

Answers to the Cholesterol and Heart Disease IQ Quiz

1. **True.** High blood cholesterol is one of the risk factors for heart disease that you can do something about. High blood pressure, cigarette smoking, diabetes, overweight, and physical inactivity are the others.

2. **False.** Although some red meat is high in saturated fat and cholesterol, which can raise your blood cholesterol, you do not need to stop eating it or any other single food. Red meat is an important source of protein, iron, and other vitamins and minerals. You should, however, cut back on the amount of saturated fat and cholesterol that you eat. One way to do this is by choosing lean cuts of meat with the fat trimmed. Another way is to watch your portion sizes and eat no more than 6 ounces of meat a day. Six ounces is about the size of two decks of playing cards.

3. **False.** A total blood cholesterol level of under 200 mg/dL is desirable and usually puts you at a lower risk for heart disease. A blood cholesterol level of 240 mg/dL is high and increases your risk of heart disease. If your cholesterol level is high, your doctor will want to check your level of LDL cholesterol ("bad" cholesterol). A high level of LDL cholesterol increases your risk of heart disease, as does a low level of HDL cholesterol ("good" cholesterol). An HDL cholesterol level below 35 mg/dL is considered a risk factor for heart disease. A total cholesterol level of 200–239 mg/dL is considered borderline-high and usually increases your risk for heart disease. All adults 20 years of age or older should have their blood cholesterol level checked at least once every 5 years.

4. **False.** Fish oils are a source of omega-3 fatty acids, which are a type of polyunsaturated fat. Fish oil supplements generally do not reduce blood cholesterol levels. Also, the effect of the long-term use of fish oil supplements is not known. However, fish is a good food choice because it is low in saturated fat.

5. **True.** Eating less fat, especially saturated fat, and cholesterol can lower your blood cholesterol level. Generally your blood cholesterol level should begin to drop a few weeks after you start on a cholesterol-lowering diet. How much your level drops depends on the amounts of saturated fat and cholesterol you used to eat, how high your blood cholesterol is, how much weight you lose if you are overweight, and how your body responds to the changes you make. Over time, you may reduce your blood cholesterol level by 10–50 mg/dL or even more.

6. **True.** Saturated fats raise your blood cholesterol level more than anything else does. So, the best way to reduce your cholesterol level is to cut back on the amount of saturated fats that you eat. These fats are found in largest amounts in animal products such as butter, cheese, whole milk, ice cream, cream, and fatty meats. They are also found in some vegetable oils—coconut, palm, and palm kernel oils.

7. **False.** Most vegetable oils—canola, corn, olive, safflower, soybean, and sunflower oils—contain mostly monounsaturated and polyunsaturated fats, which help lower blood cholesterol when used in place of saturated fats. However, a few vegetable oils—coconut, palm, and palm kernel oils—contain more saturated fat than unsaturated fat. A special kind of fat, called "trans fat," is formed when vegetable oil is hardened to become margarine or shortening, through a process called "hydrogenation." The harder the margarine or shortening, the more likely it is to contain more trans fat. Choose margarine containing liquid vegetable oil as the first ingredient.

Check Your Cholesterol and Heart Disease IQ

Just be sure to limit the total amount of any fats or oils because even those that are unsaturated are rich sources of calories.

8. True. People who have had one heart attack are at much higher risk for a second attack. Reducing blood cholesterol levels can greatly slow down (and, in some people, even reverse) the buildup of cholesterol and fat in the walls of the coronary arteries and significantly reduce the chances of a second heart attack. If you have had a heart attack or have coronary heart disease, your LDL level should be around 100 mg/dL, which is even lower than the recommended level of less than 130 mg/dL for the general population.

9. False. Children from "high-risk" families, in which a parent has high blood cholesterol (240 mg/dL or above) or in which a parent or grandparent has had heart disease at an early age (at 55 years or younger), should have their cholesterol levels tested. If a child from such a family has a cholesterol level that is high, it should be lowered under medical supervision, primarily with diet, to reduce the risk of developing heart disease as an adult. For most children, who are not from high-risk families, the best way to reduce the risk of adult heart disease is to follow a low saturated fat, low cholesterol eating pattern. All children over the age of 2 years and all adults should adopt a heart-healthy eating pattern as a principal way of reducing coronary heart disease.

10. False. Blood cholesterol levels in both men and women begin to go up around age 20. Women before menopause have levels that are lower than men of the same age. After menopause, a women's LDL cholesterol level goes up—and so her risk for heart disease increases. For both men and women, heart disease is the number one cause of death.

11. True. Food labels have been changed. Look on the nutrition label for the amount of saturated fat, total fat, cholesterol, and total calories in a serving of the product. Use this information to compare similar products. Also, look for the list of ingredients. Here, the ingredient in the greatest amount is first and the ingredient in the least amount is last. So, to choose foods low in saturated fat or total fat, go easy on products that list fats or oil first, or that list many fat and oil ingredients.

Source: National Heart, Lung, and Blood Institute (NHLBI) and National Institutes of Health (NIH). (1995, May). *Cholesterol & Heart Disease IQ* (NIH Pub. No. 95-3794). Online: http://www.nhlbi.nih.gov/health/public/heart/chol/chol_iq.htm.

Name: _____ Course Number: _____

Section: _____ Date: _____

Check Your Physical Activity and Heart Disease IQ

Directions: Test how much you know about how physical activity affects your heart. Mark each statement true or false. See how you did by checking the answers on the next page.

	True	False
1. Regular physical activity can reduce your chances of getting heart disease.	____	____
2. Most people get enough physical activity from their normal daily routine.	____	____
3. You don't have to train like a marathon runner to become more physically fit.	____	____
4. Exercise programs do not require a lot of time to be very effective.	____	____
5. People who need to lose some weight are the only ones who will benefit from regular physical activity.	____	____
6. All exercises give you the same benefits.	____	____
7. The older you are, the less active you need to be.	____	____
8. It doesn't take a lot of money or expensive equipment to become physically fit.	____	____
9. Many risks and injuries can occur with exercise.	____	____
10. You should consult a doctor before starting a physical activity program.	____	____
11. People who have had a heart attack should not start any physical activity program.	____	____
12. To help stay physically active, you should perform a variety of activities.	____	____

Answers to the Physical Activity and Heart Disease IQ Quiz

1. **True**. Heart disease is almost twice as likely to develop in inactive people. Being physically inactive is a risk factor for heart disease along with cigarette smoking, high blood pressure, high blood cholesterol, and being overweight. The more risk factors you have, the greater your chance for heart disease. Regular physical activity (even mild to moderate exercise) can reduce this risk.

2. **False**. Most Americans are very busy but not very active. Every American adult should make a habit of getting 30 minutes of low to moderate levels of physical activity daily. This includes walking, gardening, and walking up stairs. If you are inactive now, begin by doing a few minutes of activity each day. If you only do some activity every once in a while, try to work something into your routine every day.

3. **True**. Low- to moderate-intensity activities, such as pleasure walking, stair climbing, yardwork, housework, dancing, and home exercises can have both short- and long-term benefits. If you are inactive, the key is to get started. One great way is to take a walk for 10 to 15 minutes during your lunch break, or take your dog for a walk every day. At least 30 minutes of physical activity every day can help to improve your heart health.

4. **True**. It takes only a few minutes a day to become more physically active. If you don't have 30 minutes in your schedule for an exercise break, try to find two 15-minute periods or even three 10-minute periods. These exercise breaks will soon become a habit you can't live without.

5. **False**. People who are physically active experience many positive benefits. Regular physical activity gives you more energy, reduces stress, and helps you to sleep better. It helps to lower high blood pressure and improves blood cholesterol levels. Physical activity helps to tone your muscles, burns off calories to help you lose extra pounds or stay at your desirable weight, and helps control your appetite. It can also increase muscle strength, help your heart and lungs work more efficiently, and let you enjoy your life more fully.

6. **False**. Low-intensity activities—if performed daily—can have some long-term health benefits and can lower your risk of heart disease. Regular, brisk, and sustained exercise for at least 30 minutes, three to four times a week, such as brisk walking, jogging, or swimming, is necessary to improve the efficiency of your heart and lungs and burn off extra calories. These activities are called aerobic—meaning the body uses oxygen to produce the energy needed for the activity. Other activities, depending on the type, may give you other benefits such as increased flexibility or muscle strength.

7. **False**. Although we tend to become less active with age, physical activity is still important. In fact, regular physical activity in older persons increases their capacity to do everyday activities. In general, middle-aged and older people benefit from regular physical activity just as young people do. What is important, at any age, is tailoring the activity program to your own fitness level.

8. **True**. Many activities require little or no equipment. For example, brisk walking only requires a comfortable pair of walking shoes. Many communities offer free or inexpensive recreation facilities and physical activity classes. Check your shopping

malls because many of them are open early and late for people who do not wish to walk alone, in the dark, or in bad weather.

9. **False.** The most common risk in exercising is injury to the muscles and joints. Such injuries are usually caused by exercising too hard for too long, particularly if a person has been inactive. To avoid injuries, try to build up your level of activity gradually, listen to your body for warning pains, be aware of possible signs of heart problems (such as pain or pressure in the left or midchest area, left neck, shoulder, or arm during or just after exercising, or sudden light-headedness, cold sweat, pallor, or fainting), and be prepared for special weather conditions.

10. **True.** You should ask your doctor before you start (or greatly increase) your physical activity if you have a medical condition such as high blood pressure, have pains or pressure in the chest and shoulder, feel dizzy or faint, get breathless after mild exertion, are middle-aged or older and have not been physically active, or plan a vigorous activity program. If none of these apply, start slow and get moving.

11. **False.** Regular physical activity can help reduce your risk of having another heart attack. People who include regular physical activity in their lives after a heart attack improve their chances of survival and can improve how they feel and look. If you have had a heart attack, consult your doctor to be sure you are following a safe and effective exercise program that will help prevent heart pain and further damage from overexertion.

12. **True.** Pick several different activities that you like doing. You will be more likely to stay with it. Plan short-term and long-term goals. Keep a record of your progress, and check it regularly to see the progress you have made. Get your family and friends to join in. They can help keep you going.

Source: National Heart, Lung, and Blood Institute (NHLBI) and National Institutes of Health (NIH). (1996, August). *Physical Activity & Heart Disease IQ* (NIH Pub. No. 96-3795). Online: http://www.nhlbi.nih.gov/health/public/heart/obesity/phy_act.htm.

Name: _____ Course Number: _____

Section: _____ Date: _____

My Heart Disease Risk

Directions

1. Go to the online assessment tool "Your Disease Risk: The Source on Prevention" at http://www.yourdiseaserisk.wustl.edu. Here, you can find out your risk of developing heart disease in the United States and get personalized tips for preventing heart disease.

2. Click the What's your heart disease risk? link, and then click Questionnaire.

3. Is your risk low, average, or high? _____

4. Click the What makes up your risk? button, and list the factors that raise your risk and the factors that lower your risk.

Factors that raise my risk of heart disease: _____

Factors that lower my risk of heart disease: _____

Name: ───────────────────────────────── Course Number: ─────────────────

Section: ───────────────────────────────── Date: ───────────────────────

My Stroke Risk

Directions

1. Go to the online assessment tool "Your Disease Risk: The Source on Prevention" at http://www.yourdiseaserisk.wustl.edu. Here, you can find out your risk of developing a stroke in the United States and get personalized tips for preventing a stroke.

2. Click the What's your stroke risk? link, and then click Questionnaire.

3. Is your risk low, average, or high? ─────────────

4. Click the What makes up your risk? button, and list the factors that raise your risk and the factors that lower your risk.

Factors that raise my risk of stroke: ─────────────────────────

Factors that lower my risk of stroke: ─────────────────────────

Name: _____ Course Number: _____

Section: _____ Date: _____

My Diabetes Risk

Directions

1. Go to the online assessment tool "Your Disease Risk: The Source on Prevention" at http://www.yourdiseaserisk.wustl.edu. Here, you can find out your risk of developing diabetes in the United States and get personalized tips for preventing diabetes.

2. Click the What's your diabetes risk? link, and then click Questionnaire.

3. Is your risk low, average, or high? _____

4. Click the What makes up your risk? button, and list the factors that raise your risk and the factors that lower your risk.

Factors that raise my risk of diabetes: _____

Factors that lower my risk of diabetes: _____

Chapter 14: Critical Thinking Questions

Protecting Your Cardiovascular System

1. Make a list of all the six major modifiable risk factors that increase your chances of getting CVD. Which risk factors pertain to you? How can you modify or change any of these risk factors?

2. A risk factor of cardiovascular disease is family history. Family history of CVD does not guarantee that you will get the disease, and neither does it cancel out the importance of a healthy lifestyle. A family history of CVD does predispose you to the disease, so it is important for you to determine your family CVD history. Construct a family tree by listing your biological parents, siblings, grandparents (maternal and paternal), and aunts and uncles (maternal and paternal). Next to each name, list the CVD disease and the age at which it was discovered. Your family may be helpful with this activity. After completing your tree, you may want to share it with your family and discuss prevention efforts.

3. Elena is a 21-year-old college student who is very studious. Because her studies are her number one priority (she wants to go to graduate school), Elena finds it difficult to make time to maintain a healthy lifestyle, despite knowing how important it is. Although Elena is not a regular smoker, she has a tendency to smoke when under stress (studying for finals) and frequently eats nonnutritious snacks. Elena was active in high school sports, but she does not seem to find time for sports now that she is in college. As a matter of fact, she has gained about 15 pounds, although she would not be considered overweight. What can you suggest to help Elena reduce her risk of cardiovascular disease?

_____

_____

_____

_____

_____

_____

_____

_____

_____

_____

_____

_____

Critical Thinking Questions

15.1

Name: _____ Course Number: _____

Section: _____ Date: _____

Assessing Your Disease Risk

There's a lot you can do to lower your risk of cancer, heart disease, stroke, and diabetes. Take this quiz to estimate your risk of getting these diseases and highlight steps you can take to improve your health. For a more detailed estimate of your risk for specific types of cancer and other diseases, please visit http://www.yourdiseaserisk.harvard.edu.

Directions: Look at each statement. If it describes you, circle all the numbers in the boxes to the right. If it doesn't describe you, simply leave the row blank. When you're done, add the circled numbers in each column to see which disease risk category you're in.

	Cancer*	Heart Disease	Stroke	Diabetes
Tobacco use: I smoke—even sometimes.	3	3	3	1
Weight: I have gained 20 lbs or more since age 18.	1	2	1	3
Physical activity: I get less than 30 minutes of moderate activity (such as walking) on most days.	1	1	1	1
Red meat: I eat 3 or more servings of red meat per week.	1	1		
Multivitamin: I do not usually take a multivitamin.	1	1		
Fruits and vegetables: I eat fewer than 3 servings of fruits and vegetables per day.	1	1		
Whole grains: I eat fewer than 3 servings per day of whole grains (such as whole-wheat bread, brown rice, oatmeal, or whole-grain cereal).	1	1	1	1
Mono- and polyunsaturated fats: I eat oil-based salad dressing or use liquid vegetable oil for cooking 3 or fewer days per week.	1	1		
Alcohol: I average more than 1 alcoholic drink per day. (One drink is one beer, one glass of wine, or one shot of other alcohol.)	1			

* Including the most common cancers: prostate, breast, lung, and colon.

	Cancer*	Heart Disease	Stroke	Diabetes
Screening *Age 50 and over only:* I have *not* had a colonoscopy in the last 10 years.	1			
Female only: I have *not* had a Pap test in the last 3 years.	1			
Family history: I have a family history of the following diseases: (circle only those that apply from the columns at the right)	1	1	1	1
Total				

* Including the most common cancers: prostate, breast, lung, and colon.

©Copyright 2005 President and Fellows of Harvard College. Reprinted with permission of Harvard Center for Cancer Prevention, Harvard School of Public Health.

Compared to someone your age and sex, your disease risk is:

Total Points: 0–2 = Below average risk

3–4 = Average risk

5+ = Above average risk

What Your Risk Score Means

Below average disease risk. Keep up the good work. You're doing great, but it's important to stay on track. Use the quiz as an opportunity to see what makes your risk below average, and continue those healthy behaviors.

Average disease risk. Make moves to improve. You're doing many things well, but you likely have a number of steps you can take that will lower your risk even more. If you smoke, the best thing to do is stop as soon as possible. Although being "average risk" can feel comforting, try to use your score as an opportunity to target those things you can improve.

Above average disease risk. Change for the better. You have some big steps you can take to lower your risk. Tackle one thing at a time, like stopping smoking or getting more exercise, and then slowly add other healthy behaviors. Also, talk to your doctor about your risk factors to see if you might need to take special steps, like extra screening or medications, to protect yourself further.

Name: _____ Course Number: _____

Section: _____ Date: _____

My Cancer Risk

Directions

1. Go to the online assessment tool "Your Disease Risk: The Source on Prevention" at http://www.yourdiseaserisk.wustl.edu. Here, you can find out your risk of developing cancer in the United States and get personalized tips for preventing cancer.

2. Click on "What Is Your Cancer Risk?" and choose three different cancers (bladder, breast, cervical, colon, kidney, lung, melanoma, ovarian, pancreatic, prostate, stomach, uterine) and assess risk by completing the accompanying questionnaire.

3. Is your risk low, average, or high for _____ cancer? _____

4. Click on "What makes up your risk?" and list the factors that raise your risk and the factors that lower your risk.

   Factors that raise my risk of _____ cancer: _____

   Factors that lower my risk of _____ cancer: _____

5. Is your risk low, average, or high for _____ cancer? _____

6. Click on "What makes up your risk?" and list the factors that raise your risk and the factors that lower your risk.

   Factors that raise my risk of _____ cancer: _____

   Factors that lower my risk of _____ cancer: _____

7. Is your risk low, average, or high for _____ cancer? _____

8. Click on "What makes up your risk?" and list the factors that raise your risk and the factors that lower your risk.

   Factors that raise my risk of _____ cancer: _____

   Factors that lower my risk of_____ cancer: _____

9. Is your risk low, average, or high for _____ cancer? _____

Name: _____   Course Number: _____

Section: _____   Date: _____

Chapter 15: Critical Thinking Questions

Reducing Your Cancer Risk

1. Make a list of all the modifiable risk factors that increase your chance of getting cancer. Order the list from the highest to lowest risk. Which risk factors pertain to you? How can you modify or change these risk factors?

2. Family history is a risk factor for cancer. A family history of cancer does not guarantee that you will get the disease, and neither does it cancel out the importance of a healthy lifestyle (not smoking, good dietary habits, and regular physical activity). A family history of cancer does predispose you to the disease; therefore, it is important for you to determine your family cancer history. Construct a family tree by listing your biological parents, siblings, grandparents (maternal and paternal), and aunts and uncles (maternal and paternal). A sample family cancer history diagram is shown here. Next to each name, list the type of cancer and the age at which it was discovered. Your family may be helpful with this activity. After completing your tree, you may want to share it with your family and discuss prevention efforts (include cancer screenings and early detection methods).

3. Do you have any family members or friends like Katrina who would like to quit smoking? If yes, go online to the American Cancer Society website and search for ways to quit smoking. After completing this activity, sit down and share the information with the individual trying to quit smoking.

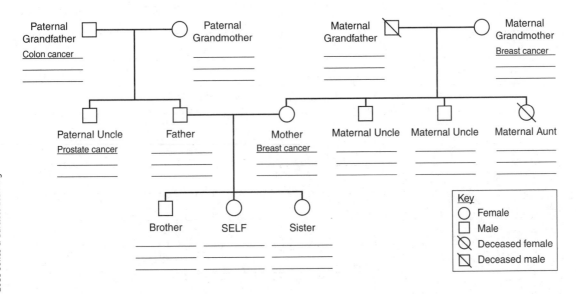

Name: ——————————————————————— Course Number: ———————————————

Section: ——————————————————————— Date: ———————————————————

Discussing Sexual Issues

In this chapter, you will be discussing information and issues related to sexual relationships. Sometimes certain sexual acts can be difficult to discuss in a group.

1. What do you think makes it difficult to discuss sexual acts in a group?

———————————————————————————————————————

———————————————————————————————————————

———————————————————————————————————————

———————————————————————————————————————

———————————————————————————————————————

2. Share some of your reasons with a small group of students. List the issues that your entire group identified.

———————————————————————————————————————

———————————————————————————————————————

———————————————————————————————————————

———————————————————————————————————————

———————————————————————————————————————

3. How might discussions be made less difficult? Are there guidelines that the class can follow to promote rich discussion?

———————————————————————————————————————

———————————————————————————————————————

———————————————————————————————————————

———————————————————————————————————————

———————————————————————————————————————

Name: _____ Course Number: _____

Section: _____ Date: _____

An Ounce of Prevention

Conduct an informal interview of students (not from this class) regarding their feelings about the pros and cons of the following STI safer sex techniques for college students.

	Pros	Cons
Abstinence		
Delaying having sex with a potential partner until you know him/her well enough to assess risk and discuss STI concerns		
Long-term monogamous sexual relationship with an uninfected partner		
Using a latex condom, dental dam, female condom, or other barrier while performing sexual acts		
Limiting the number of concurrent sexual partners		
Refraining from the use of alcohol and other drugs before having sex		

Based on the information you have gathered from your peers, what do you recommend as an effective strategy for college students to reduce the risk of contracting sexually transmitted infections? Why?

_____

_____

_____

_____

Name: ———————————————————— Course Number: ——————————

Section: ———————————————————— Date: ——————————

Can You Be Assertive When You Need to Be?

To take the necessary actions to prevent contracting a sexually transmitted infection, you will have to be assertive. That is, you will need to resist pressure to engage in sexual activity if you choose not to, and you will need to insist on the use of a condom and other safer-sex precautions if you do decide to engage in sex. Do you have assertiveness skills? To find out, write an assertive response to each of the following situations.

1. You are on a date and your partner insists on engaging in a sexual activity that you decide is not for you at that time. You say:

———————————————————————————————

———————————————————————————————

———————————————————————————————

———————————————————————————————

2. Your partner argues that condoms diminish the sensation. You respond by saying:

———————————————————————————————

———————————————————————————————

———————————————————————————————

———————————————————————————————

3. Your partner states that she or he has been tested for STIs and the test was negative. Therefore, there are no reasons for using safer-sex techniques. You respond by saying:

———————————————————————————————

———————————————————————————————

———————————————————————————————

———————————————————————————————

To Be Assertive, You Need To

- Specify the behavior or situation to which the statement refers.

- Relate your feelings about that situation.

- Suggest a remedy or what you would prefer to see occur.

- Identify the consequences of the change; what will happen if it occurs and what will happen if it does not occur.

  Now, check your responses and revise them to be consistent with these assertiveness principles.

Source: J.S. Greenberg, C.E. Bruess, & S. Conklin. (2007). *Exploring the Dimensions of Human Sexuality*, 3rd ed. Sudbury, MA: Jones & Bartlett, 604–605.

Name: _____ Course Number: _____

Section: _____ Date: _____

Chapter 16: Critical Thinking Questions

Preventing Sexually Transmitted Infections

1. Jeremy and Christina have chosen to abstain from sexual intercourse. Describe for yourself the pros and cons of sexual abstinence. Have you been able to discuss your thoughts about sexuality with your current partner?

2. As more and more people become infected with HIV, more students attending universities and colleges are infected with HIV. Many universities have residence halls with living quarters that accommodate two to four people of the same gender. Is it necessary for universities to notify students in a residence hall if a person living there is HIV-positive? If not, why not?

3. Herpes is a sexually transmitted infection that lasts a lifetime; however, herpes can be managed with medication. Explain, in detail, how you would go about telling your new partner that you have herpes.

4. You and your best college friend are talking, and your friend confides to you that about 2 months ago he may have had sexual intercourse with someone who could be HIV-positive, but your friend is not having any symptoms. What advice would you give him?

_____

_____

_____

_____

_____

_____

_____

_____

_____

_____

_____

_____

Critical Thinking Questions

Name: ———————————————————— Course Number: ————————————

Section: ———————————————————— Date: ————————————————

Diet and Activity Records

The diet and activity records in this appendix provide enough forms to record your intakes and expenditures for an entire week. The forms for each day are placed together. Use as many forms as necessary to complete your assigment.

Diet Record Day 1

Name: _____   Date: _____

☐ Weekday
☐ Weekend Day

Eating Behavior Diary

Time of Day	M, S, or B[1]	H[2] (0–3)	Location	Activity While Eating	Others Present	Time Spent Eating	Food Eaten and Quantity (describe preparation, variety, etc., as needed)	Reason for Choice[3]	Helpings (0,–,+)[4]	S[5] (0–3)

[1] Indicate whether the eating/drinking event was a meal, a snack, or a beverage.

[2] Degree of hunger: 0 = not at all hungry; 1 = slightly hungry; 2 = moderately hungry; 3 = very hungry. If only a beverage was consumed, apply the scale to the degree of thirst.

[3] Reason for food choice: Examples include taste, habit, convenience, health, weight control, hunger, thirst, stress, comfort, offered to me, and so on.

[4] Helpings: 0 = ate all that you were first served but not more; – = ate less than what you were served; + = ate more than you were originally served.

[5] Degree of satiation: 0 = not at all satisfied; 1 = still a little hungry; 2 = satisfied and comfortable; 3 = very full.

Eating Behavior Diary

Time of Day	M, S, or B[1]	H[2] (0–3)	Location	Activity While Eating	Others Present	Time Spent Eating	Food Eaten and Quantity (describe preparation, variety, etc., as needed)	Reason for Choice[3]	Helpings (0,–,+)[4]	S[5] (0–3)

[1] Indicate whether the eating/drinking event was a meal, a snack, or a beverage.

[2] Degree of hunger: 0 = not at all hungry; 1 = slightly hungry; 2 = moderately hungry; 3 = very hungry. If only a beverage was consumed, apply the scale to the degree of thirst.

[3] Reason for food choice: Examples include taste, habit, convenience, health, weight control, hunger, thirst, stress, comfort, offered to me, and so on.

[4] Helpings: 0 = ate all that you were first served but not more; – = ate less than what you were served; + = ate more than you were originally served.

[5] Degree of satiation: 0 = not at all satisfied; 1 = still a little hungry; 2 = satisfied and comfortable; 3 = very full.

Activity Record Day 1

Name: _____ Date: _____

☐ Weekday
☐ Weekend Day

Activity Record			
Time of Day	Duration (Minutes)	Description of Activity	Level of Activity

Activity Record			
Time of Day	Duration (Minutes)	Description of Activity	Level of Activity

Total Duration: _____ (must equal 1440 minutes for the entire 24-hour period)

Diet Record Day 2

Name: _____ Date: _____ ☐ Weekday
☐ Weekend Day

Eating Behavior Diary

Time of Day	M, S, or B[1]	H[2] (0–3)	Location	Activity While Eating	Others Present	Time Spent Eating	Food Eaten and Quantity (describe preparation, variety, etc., as needed)	Reason for Choice[3]	Helpings (0,–,+)[4]	S[5] (0–3)

[1] Indicate whether the eating/drinking event was a meal, a snack, or a beverage.

[2] Degree of hunger: 0 = not at all hungry; 1 = slightly hungry; 2 = moderately hungry; 3 = very hungry. If only a beverage was consumed, apply the scale to the degree of thirst.

[3] Reason for food choice: Examples include taste, habit, convenience, health, weight control, hunger, thirst, stress, comfort, offered to me, and so on.

[4] Helpings: 0 = ate all that you were first served but not more; – = ate less than what you were served; + = ate more than you were originally served.

[5] Degree of satiation: 0 = not at all satisfied; 1 = still a little hungry; 2 = satisfied and comfortable; 3 = very full.

Eating Behavior Diary

Time of Day	M, S, or B[1]	H[2] (0–3)	Location	Activity While Eating	Others Present	Time Spent Eating	Food Eaten and Quantity (describe preparation, variety, etc., as needed)	Reason for Choice[3]	Helpings (0,–,+)[4]	S[5] (0–3)

[1] Indicate whether the eating/drinking event was a meal, a snack, or a beverage.

[2] Degree of hunger: 0 = not at all hungry; 1 = slightly hungry; 2 = moderately hungry; 3 = very hungry. If only a beverage was consumed, apply the scale to the degree of thirst.

[3] Reason for food choice: Examples include taste, habit, convenience, health, weight control, hunger, thirst, stress, comfort, offered to me, and so on.

[4] Helpings: 0 = ate all that you were first served but not more; – = ate less than what you were served; + = ate more than you were originally served.

[5] Degree of satiation: 0 = not at all satisfied; 1 = still a little hungry; 2 = satisfied and comfortable; 3 = very full.

Activity Record Day 2

Name: _____ Date: _____

□ Weekday
□ Weekend Day

Activity Record			
Time of Day	Duration (Minutes)	Description of Activity	Level of Activity

Activity Record

Time of Day	Duration (Minutes)	Description of Activity	Level of Activity

Total Duration: _____ (must equal 1440 minutes for the entire 24-hour period)

Diet Record Day 3

Name: _____

Date: _____

☐ Weekday
☐ Weekend Day

Eating Behavior Diary

Time of Day	M, S, or B[1]	H[2] (0–3)	Location	Activity While Eating	Others Present	Time Spent Eating	Food Eaten and Quantity (describe preparation, variety, etc. as needed)	Reason for Choice[3]	Helpings (0,−,+)[4]	S[5] (0–3)

[1] Indicate whether the eating/drinking event was a meal, a snack, or a beverage.

[2] Degree of hunger: 0 = not at all hungry; 1 = slightly hungry; 2 = moderately hungry; 3 = very hungry. If only a beverage was consumed, apply the scale to the degree of thirst.

[3] Reason for food choice: Examples include taste, habit, convenience, health, weight control, hunger, thirst, stress, comfort, offered to me, and so on.

[4] Helpings: 0 = ate all that you were first served but not more; − = ate less than what you were served; + = ate more than you were originally served.

[5] Degree of satiation: 0 = not at all satisfied; 1 = still a little hungry; 2 = satisfied and comfortable; 3 = very full.

Eating Behavior Diary

Time of Day	M, S, or B[1]	H[2] (0–3)	Location	Activity While Eating	Others Present	Time Spent Eating	Food Eaten and Quantity (describe preparation, variety, etc., as needed)	Reason for Choice[3]	Helpings (0, −, +)[4]	S[5] (0–3)

[1] Indicate whether the eating/drinking event was a meal, a snack, or a beverage.

[2] Degree of hunger: 0 = not at all hungry; 1 = slightly hungry; 2 = moderately hungry; 3 = very hungry. If only a beverage was consumed, apply the scale to the degree of thirst.

[3] Reason for food choice: Examples include taste, habit, convenience, health, weight control, hunger, thirst, stress, comfort, offered to me, and so on.

[4] Helpings: 0 = ate all that you were first served but not more; − = ate less than what you were served; + = ate more than you were originally served.

[5] Degree of satiation: 0 = not at all satisfied; 1 = still a little hungry; 2 = satisfied and comfortable; 3 = very full.

Activity Record Day 3

Name: _____ Date: _____

☐ Weekday
☐ Weekend Day

Activity Record

Time of Day	Duration (Minutes)	Description of Activity	Level of Activity

	Activity Record		
Time of Day	Duration (Minutes)	Description of Activity	Level of Activity

Total Duration: _____ (must equal 1440 minutes for the entire 24-hour period)

Diet Record Day 4

Name: _____   Date: _____

☐ Weekday
☐ Weekend Day

Eating Behavior Diary

Time of Day	M, S, or B[1]	H[2] (0–3)	Location	Activity While Eating	Others Present	Time Spent Eating	Food Eaten and Quantity (describe preparation, variety, etc., as needed)	Reason for Choice[3]	Helpings (0,−,+)[4]	S[5] (0–3)

[1] Indicate whether the eating/drinking event was a meal, a snack, or a beverage.

[2] Degree of hunger: 0 = not at all hungry; 1 = slightly hungry; 2 = moderately hungry; 3 = very hungry. If only a beverage was consumed, apply the scale to the degree of thirst.

[3] Reason for food choice: Examples include taste, habit, convenience, health, weight control, hunger, thirst, stress, comfort, offered to me, and so on.

[4] Helpings: 0 = ate all that you were first served but not more; − = ate less than what you were served; + = ate more than you were originally served.

[5] Degree of satiation: 0 = not at all satisfied; 1 = still a little hungry; 2 = satisfied and comfortable; 3 = very full.

Diet and Activity Records

Eating Behavior Diary

Time of Day	M, S, or B[1]	H[2] (0–3)	Location	Activity While Eating	Others Present	Time Spent Eating	Food Eaten and Quantity (describe preparation, variety, etc., as needed)	Reason for Choice[3]	Helpings (0,–,+)[4]	S[5] (0–3)

[1] Indicate whether the eating/drinking event was a meal, a snack, or a beverage.

[2] Degree of hunger: 0 = not at all hungry; 1 = slightly hungry; 2 = moderately hungry; 3 = very hungry. If only a beverage was consumed, apply the scale to the degree of thirst.

[3] Reason for food choice: Examples include taste, habit, convenience, health, weight control, hunger, thirst, stress, comfort, offered to me, and so on.

[4] Helpings: 0 = ate all that you were first served but not more; – = ate less than what you were served; + = ate more than you were originally served.

[5] Degree of satiation: 0 = not at all satisfied; 1 = still a little hungry; 2 = satisfied and comfortable; 3 = very full.

Activity Record Day 4

Name: _____   Date: _____

☐ Weekday
☐ Weekend Day

Activity Record

Time of Day	Duration (Minutes)	Description of Activity	Level of Activity

Activity Record			
Time of Day	Duration (Minutes)	Description of Activity	Level of Activity

Total Duration: _____ (must equal 1440 minutes for the entire 24-hour period)

Diet Record Day 5

Name: _____

Date: _____

☐ Weekday
☐ Weekend Day

Eating Behavior Diary

Time of Day	M, S, or B[1]	H[2] (0–3)	Location	Activity While Eating	Others Present	Time Spent Eating	Food Eaten and Quantity (describe preparation, variety, etc., as needed)	Reason for Choice[3]	Helpings (0,−,+)[4]	S[5] (0–3)

[1] Indicate whether the eating/drinking event was a meal, a snack, or a beverage.

[2] Degree of hunger: 0 = not at all hungry; 1 = slightly hungry; 2 = moderately hungry; 3 = very hungry. If only a beverage was consumed, apply the scale to the degree of thirst.

[3] Reason for food choice: Examples include taste, habit, convenience, health, weight control, hunger, thirst, stress, comfort, offered to me, and so on.

[4] Helpings: 0 = ate all that you were first served but not more; − = ate less than what you were served; + = ate more than you were originally served.

[5] Degree of satiation: 0 = not at all satisfied; 1 = still a little hungry; 2 = satisfied and comfortable; 3 = very full.

Eating Behavior Diary

Time of Day	M, S, or B[1]	H[2] (0–3)	Location	Activity While Eating	Others Present	Time Spent Eating	Food Eaten and Quantity (describe preparation, variety, etc., as needed)	Reason for Choice[3]	Helpings (0,–,+)[4]	S[5] (0–3)

[1] Indicate whether the eating/drinking event was a meal, a snack, or a beverage.

[2] Degree of hunger: 0 = not at all hungry; 1 = slightly hungry; 2 = moderately hungry; 3 = very hungry. If only a beverage was consumed, apply the scale to the degree of thirst.

[3] Reason for food choice: Examples include taste, habit, convenience, health, weight control, hunger, thirst, stress, comfort, offered to me, and so on.

[4] Helpings: 0 = ate all that you were first served but not more; – = ate less than what you were served; + = ate more than you were originally served.

[5] Degree of satiation: 0 = not at all satisfied; 1 = still a little hungry; 2 = satisfied and comfortable; 3 = very full.

Activity Record Day 5

Name: _____   Date: _____

☐ Weekday
☐ Weekend Day

Activity Record

Time of Day	Duration (Minutes)	Description of Activity	Level of Activity

		Activity Record	
Time of Day	Duration (Minutes)	Description of Activity	Level of Activity

Total Duration: _____ (must equal 1440 minutes for the entire 24-hour period)

Diet Record Day 6

Name: _____ Date: _____

☐ Weekday
☐ Weekend Day

Eating Behavior Diary

Time of Day	M, S, or B[1]	H[2] (0–3)	Location	Activity While Eating	Others Present	Time Spent Eating	Food Eaten and Quantity (describe preparation, variety, etc., as needed)	Reason for Choice[3]	Helpings (0,–,+)[4]	S[5] (0–3)

[1] Indicate whether the eating/drinking event was a meal, a snack, or a beverage.

[2] Degree of hunger: 0 = not at all hungry; 1 = slightly hungry; 2 = moderately hungry; 3 = very hungry. If only a beverage was consumed, apply the scale to the degree of thirst.

[3] Reason for food choice: Examples include taste, habit, convenience, health, weight control, hunger, thirst, stress, comfort, offered to me, and so on.

[4] Helpings: 0 = ate all that you were first served but not more; – = ate less than what you were served; + = ate more than you were originally served.

[5] Degree of satiation: 0 = not at all satisfied; 1 = still a little hungry; 2 = satisfied and comfortable; 3 = very full.

Eating Behavior Diary

Time of Day	M, S, or B[1]	H[2] (0–3)	Location	Activity While Eating	Others Present	Time Spent Eating	Food Eaten and Quantity (describe preparation, variety, etc., as needed)	Reason for Choice[3]	Helpings (0,–,+)[4]	S[5] (0–3)

[1] Indicate whether the eating/drinking event was a meal, a snack, or a beverage.

[2] Degree of hunger: 0 = not at all hungry; 1 = slightly hungry; 2 = moderately hungry; 3 = very hungry. If only a beverage was consumed, apply the scale to the degree of thirst.

[3] Reason for food choice: Examples include taste, habit, convenience, health, weight control, hunger, thirst, stress, comfort, offered to me, and so on.

[4] Helpings: 0 = ate all that you were first served but not more; – = ate less than what you were served; + = ate more than you were originally served.

[5] Degree of satiation: 0 = not at all satisfied; 1 = still a little hungry; 2 = satisfied and comfortable; 3 = very full.

Activity Record Day 6

Name: _____   Date: _____

☐ Weekday
☐ Weekend Day

Activity Record

Time of Day	Duration (Minutes)	Description of Activity	Level of Activity

	Activity Record		
Time of Day	Duration (Minutes)	Description of Activity	Level of Activity

Total Duration: _____ (must equal 1440 minutes for the entire 24-hour period)

Diet Record Day 7

Name: _____

Date: _____

☐ Weekday
☐ Weekend Day

Eating Behavior Diary

Time of Day	M, S, or B[1]	H[2] (0-3)	Location	Activity While Eating	Others Present	Time Spent Eating	Food Eaten and Quantity (describe preparation, variety, etc., as needed)	Reason for Choice[3]	Helpings (0,–,+)[4]	S[5] (0-3)

[1] Indicate whether the eating/drinking event was a meal, a snack, or a beverage.

[2] Degree of hunger: 0 = not at all hungry; 1 = slightly hungry; 2 = moderately hungry; 3 = very hungry. If only a beverage was consumed, apply the scale to the degree of thirst.

[3] Reason for food choice: Examples include taste, habit, convenience, health, weight control, hunger, thirst, stress, comfort, offered to me, and so on.

[4] Helpings: 0 = ate all that you were first served but not more; – = ate less than what you were served; + = ate more than you were originally served.

[5] Degree of satiation: 0 = not at all satisfied; 1 = still a little hungry; 2 = satisfied and comfortable; 3 = very full.

Eating Behavior Diary

Time of Day	M, S, or B[1]	H[2] (0–3)	Location	Activity While Eating	Others Present	Time Spent Eating	Food Eaten and Quantity (describe preparation, variety, etc., as needed)	Reason for Choice[3]	Helpings (0,–,+)[4]	S[5] (0–3)

[1] Indicate whether the eating/drinking event was a meal, a snack, or a beverage.

[2] Degree of hunger: 0 = not at all hungry; 1 = slightly hungry; 2 = moderately hungry; 3 = very hungry. If only a beverage was consumed, apply the scale to the degree of thirst.

[3] Reason for food choice: Examples include taste, habit, convenience, health, weight control, hunger, thirst, stress, comfort, offered to me, and so on.

[4] Helpings: 0 = ate all that you were first served but not more; – = ate less than what you were served; + = ate more than you were originally served.

[5] Degree of satiation: 0 = not at all satisfied; 1 = still a little hungry; 2 = satisfied and comfortable; 3 = very full.

Activity Record Day 7

Name: _____ Date: _____

☐ Weekday
☐ Weekend Day

Activity Record

Time of Day	Duration (Minutes)	Description of Activity	Level of Activity

Activity Record			
Time of Day	Duration (Minutes)	Description of Activity	Level of Activity

Total Duration: _____ (must equal 1440 minutes for the entire 24-hour period)

Name: _____ Course Number: _____

Section: _____ Date: _____

Growth Charts: Stature-for-Age and Weight-for-Age Percentiles for Children and Teenagers

For children and teenagers, healthy weight status is defined differently than it is for adults. Because children and teenagers are still growing, boys and girls develop at different rates. The body mass index (BMI) for a child aged 2 to 20 years is determined by comparing his or her weight and height against the appropriate growth chart that account for age and gender. (See the Centers for Disease Control and Prevention's [CDC] growth charts for boys and girls on the following pages).

Tracking Changes in BMI-for-Age

1. Select the appropriate chart.

2. Calculate BMI using the formula on the growth chart or using the online BMI percentile calculator available at http://apps.nccd.cdc.gov/dnpabmi/Calculator.aspx.

3. Plot the BMI percentile number obtained from the formula or calculator against the child's age.

4. Use the following table to interpret the results.

BMI Percentile-for-Age	Suggests the Child/Teenager Is
At or over the 95th percentile	Obese
Between the 85th and 95th percentiles	Overweight
Between 15th and 85th percentiles	Probably at a healthy weight
Between 5th and 15th percentiles	Possibly at risk for underweight
Under the 5th percentile	Underweight

5. Every few months, recalculate the child or teen's BMI percentile and plot on the chart.

2 to 20 years: Boys
Stature-for-Age and Weight-for-Age Percentiles

NAME _____

RECORD # _____

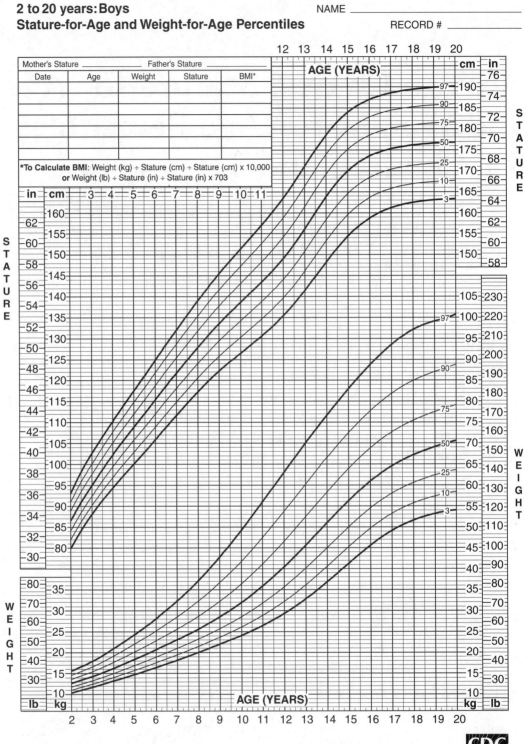

Source: Developed by the National Center for Health Statistics in collaboration with the National Center for Chronic Disease Prevention and Health Promotion (2000). Online: http://www.cdc.gov/growthcharts.

Growth Charts: Stature-for-Age and Weight-for-Age Percentiles for Children and Teenagers

2 to 20 years: Girls
Stature-for-Age and Weight-for-Age Percentiles

NAME _____

RECORD # _____

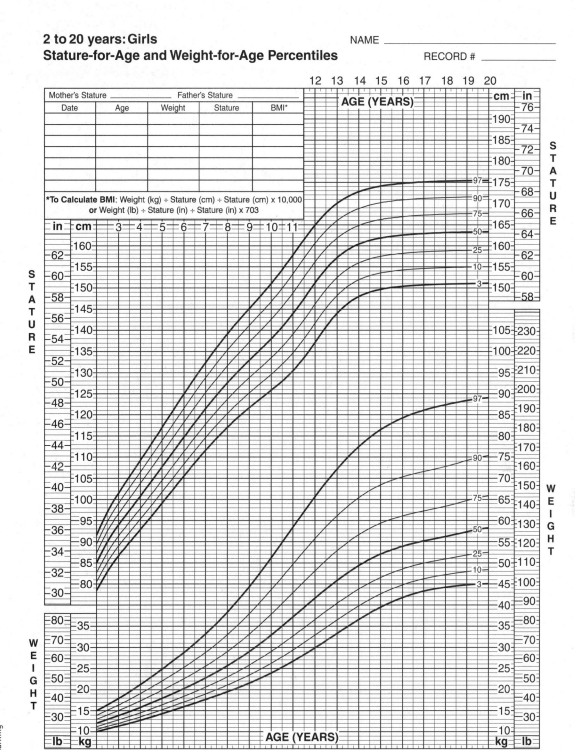

Source: Developed by the National Center for Health Statistics in collaboration with the National Center for Chronic Disease Prevention and Health Promotion (2000). Online: http://www.cdc.gov/growthcharts.